THE DASH DIET COOKBOOK

---

90 QUICK & EASY LOW SODIUM RECIPES TO LOWER BLOOD PRESSURE. | IMPROVE YOUR HEALTH.

PAMELA KENDRICK

CONTENTS

Introduction   vii

BREAKFAST

1. Scallions Omelette   3
2. Overnight Refrigerated Oatmeal   4
3. Apple Porridge   5
4. Healthy Buckwheat Pancakes   7
5. Banana Bread   9
6. Asparagus Omelette   11
7. Mushroom Spinach Frittata   12
8. Eggs on Toast   14
9. Sweet Yogurt with Figs   16
10. Green Smoothie   17
11. Quinoa Bread   18
12. Artichoke Eggs   20
13. Muesli Bars   21
14. Sweet Potato Toast   23
15. Cinnamon and Coconut Porridge   25
16. Baking Powder Biscuits   27
17. Almond Butter Banana Chocolate Smoothie   29
18. Avocado Toast with Smoked Trout   30
19. Crunchy Flax and Almond Crackers   32
20. Grape Yogurt   34

LUNCH

21. Stir-Fry Rice with Chicken   37
22. Spinach and Beef Meatballs   39
23. Faux Mac and Cheese   40
24. Purple Potato Soup   42
25. Turkey Lettuce Wrap   44
26. Easy Salmon Steaks   46
27. Chicken and Carrot Stew   48
28. Leeks Soup   49

29. Pistachio Mint Pesto Pasta — 51
30. Lamb Curry with Tomatoes and Spinach — 53
31. Zucchini Zoodles with Chicken and Basil — 55
32. Indian Chicken Stew — 57
33. Golden Eggplant Fries — 59
34. Cauliflower Lunch Salad — 61
35. Trout Parcel — 63
36. Spinach Pork Cubes — 65
37. Tilapia Casserole — 66
38. Balsamic Vinegar Steak — 68
39. Shrimp with Asparagus — 69
40. Traditional Black Bean Chili — 71

DINNER

41. Paprika Lamb Chops — 75
42. Shrimp Cocktail — 76
43. Beef and Onion Stew — 78
44. Shrimp with White Beans and Feta — 80
45. Mussels and Chickpea Soup — 82
46. Walnuts and Asparagus Delight — 84
47. Quinoa and Scallops Salad — 85
48. Fish Stew — 87
49. Turkey breast with Coconut and Zucchini — 89
50. Creamy Pumpkin Pasta — 91
51. Tasty Roasted Broccoli — 93
52. Lime Shrimp and Kale — 94
53. Chicken Salsa — 95
54. Vegetarian Lasagna — 96
55. Carrot Cakes — 98
56. Chipotle Lettuce Chicken — 99
57. Vegan Chili — 101
58. Fruited Quinoa Salad — 102
59. Chunky Tomatoes — 104
60. Cauliflower Bread Stick — 105

SNACKS

61. Avocado Guacamole — 109
62. Savoury Stuffed Mushrooms — 110
63. Peas & Feta Sandwich — 112

64. Crusted Chicken with Dipping Sauce	113
65. Yogurt & Banana Bowl	115
66. Zucchini Sticks	116
67. Yogurt & Dried Fruit Bars	118
68. Salt-Free Pickles	120
69. Oatmeal Cookies	122
70. Cheesy Popcorn	124
71. Roasted Harissa Carrots	126
72. Chocolate Coconut Bombs	128
73. Kale Chips	129
74. Apple Dumplings	130
75. Roasted Chickpeas	132

DESSERTS

76. Frozen Mango Treat	137
77. Pumpkin with Chia Seeds Pudding	138
78. Grilled Pineapple Strips	140
79. Peach Sorbet	142
80. Choco Banana Cake	143
81. Herbed Ground Chicken	145
82. Zesty Zucchini Muffins	147
83. Mango Rice Pudding	149
84. Chicken Meatloaf	151
85. Blueberry Oat Muffins	153
86. Raspberry Peach Pancake	155
87. Turkey & Beans Lettuce Wraps	157
88. Banana Bread	159
89. Poached Pears	161
90. Strawberry Bruschetta	163

Conclusion   165

Copyright 2021 by Pamela Kendrick. All rights reserved.

The content contained within this book may not be reproduced, duplicated or transmitted without direct written permission from the author or the publisher.

Under no circumstances will any blame or legal responsibility be held against the publisher, or author, for any damages, reparation, or monetary loss due to the information contained within this book. Either directly or indirectly.

Legal Notice:

This book is copyright protected. This book is only for personal use. You cannot amend, distribute, sell, use, quote or paraphrase any part, or the content within this book, without the consent of the author or publisher.

Disclaimer Notice:

Please note the information contained within this document is for educational and entertainment purposes only. All effort has been executed to present accurate, up-to-date, and reliable, complete information. No warranties of any kind are declared or implied. Readers acknowledge that the author is not engaging in the rendering of legal, financial, medical or professional advice. The content within this book has been derived from various sources. Please consult a licensed professional before attempting any techniques outlined in this book.

By reading this document, the reader agrees that under no circumstances is the author responsible for any losses, direct or indirect, which are incurred as a result of the use of the information contained within this document, including, but not limited to, errors, omissions, or inaccuracies.

INTRODUCTION

Over time, there has been a rapid rise in the number of people living with high blood pressure. This number doubled up in the last decade, which is now seen as an epidemic that needs to be addressed.

There are many ways of addressing this problem, but one way is by reducing the amount of sodium in one's diet. The DASH diet can help to lower the amount consumed, which is a clear alternative step in preventing high blood pressure.

The body requires sodium to function properly. It is a mineral that is essential for many different parts of the human body. It also plays a vital role in controlling fluids in the human body, and you will often hear that it can keep you hydrated.

Although sodium is an essential component of our health, there are adverse effects associated with excessive sodium consumption and its negative consequences on our health.

The heart is affected by sodium in the blood, which leads to high blood pressure. To help lower your blood pressure, you need to reduce your intake of sodium through the introduction of the DASH diet.

The carotid artery, which helps to supply the brain with

Introduction

oxygenated blood, also gets affected by high sodium levels, which increases the risk of stroke.

Sodium can also cause fluid retention, and some people may look puffy around their eyes, chest, and hands when they have too much sodium in their system.

Adequate sodium intake to prevent this from happening is crucial, especially for those that are at risk of these medical conditions.

How much sodium you should consume depends on your age and lifestyle. It is recommended that if you do not have a history of high blood pressure, then you should try to consume around 2000mg of sodium a day. This means that some of your favourite foods will be cut out or reduced to keep your sodium intake relatively low.

Nevertheless, if you have a history of high blood pressure (hypertension), your daily intake will be lower. It is recommended that you consume around 1500mg of sodium a day or lower depending on your medical condition.

The best way to prevent further complications caused by sodium is by reducing the intake to as low as possible, and this is where the DASH diet comes in.

THE DASH DIET

Many people have been suffering from high blood pressure, body fat, heart disease, and other diseases. The DASH diet provides a solution to such a problem by increasing stamina and endurance

The DASH diet is a diet to lower the amount of cholesterol circulating in the blood, which leads to reducing the risk of coronary artery disease.

The goal of the DASH diet is to encourage eating of foods with lower sodium while boosting the ratio of your diet to 70 % healthy foods such as lean protein, fruits, veggies, and bran. The other 30 per cent of your diet should be from carbohydrates that are low in saturated fat while being high in fibre like oatmeal which can lower cholesterol levels and help prevent heart disease.

WHAT IS THE DASH DIET?

Introduction

Dietary Approaches to Stop Hypertension which is popularly known as the DASH diet is a complicated diet that focuses on matching your intake of food with your body's daily needs. It was formed by the National Heart, Lung, and Blood Institute (NHLBI) at the National Institutes of Health (NIH) in 1996. The purpose of this diet is to lower blood pressure levels in people over age 18 who have high blood pressure or pre-hypertension.

The DASH diet is based on the understanding that foods and beverages can raise one's blood pressure. It emphasizes eating plenty of fruits and vegetables, along with a medically approved monounsaturated fat (olive oil, canola oil), three servings of low-fat or fat-free dairy products (one serving is one cup or eight ounces), and fish. The goal of the DASH diet is to reduce the amount of salt you eat; it recommends limiting sodium intake to 2,400 milligrams per day or less.

To prevent high blood pressure, the DASH diet also recommends limiting your intake of fats and sweets, such as sugar-containing soft drinks, cakes, and cookies. It recommends limiting your daily intake of total fat to less than 25 per cent of your calories (this is lower than the 30 per cent limit recommended by many nutritionists) and eating no more than 7 teaspoons of added sugar per day.

A vital part of the DASH diet is weight control and physical activity. According to the Dietary Guidelines for Americans, you should consume a minimum of 30 minutes of moderate-intensity exercise (such as walking) on most, preferably all, days of the week. The goal is to have at least 150 minutes of moderate-intensity physical activity per week.

It does not necessitate any special foods or ingredients. It emphasizes lower fat and sodium foods and that contain monounsaturated fat, omega-3 fatty acids, and potassium. It encourages you to eat lean meats, pasta, fruits, and vegetables. It recommends that you eat at least three meals a day and have healthy snacks between meals.

The DASH diet also stresses the importance of eating a diet with a balanced mix of the nutrients found in food. This includes

Introduction

bread and cereals, fruits and vegetables, and dairy products. It also recommends that you eat foods that provide vitamins and minerals (such as vitamin C, folate, calcium and potassium) and avoid high dietary cholesterol. The DASH diet is only for adults with high blood pressure and high blood pressure risk factors.

BENEFITS OF THE DASH DIET

The DASH Diet is considered to help lose weight by eating foods that will lower blood pressure. It contains a diet rich in foods with potassium, calcium, and magnesium. The body requests all of these nutrients to function properly and regulate your blood pressure. The plan also emphasizes reducing sodium intake because it's known as the silent killer, causing high blood pressure and other cardiovascular problems. Eating low-fat dairy products is encouraged because they are filling without adding a lot of calories.

The diet influences the body in numerous ways.
- Weight loss
- Improved cholesterol levels
- Better blood pressure readings
- More energy

Weight Loss

The DASH diet emphases lowering your blood pressure, which is one of the main medical benefits of this diet. This in turn reduces stress levels, and you end up having more energy throughout the day. This means you will not feel lethargic after meals due to blood sugar crashes. The key to weight loss with the DASH Diet is to avoid sugar and refined carbohydrates and stick with complex carbohydrates. It is one of the top recommended diets for those looking for an alternative lifestyle.

Improved Cholesterol Levels

The DASH diet is an excellent way of lowering cholesterol levels without compromising the intake of nutrients and calories. It is also one of my top recommended diets for those looking for an alternative lifestyle. The DASH diet focuses on lowering your blood pressure, which is one of the main medical benefits of this diet. This in turn reduces stress levels, and you end up having more energy throughout the day. This means you will not feel lethargic after meals due to blood sugar crashes. The key to weight loss with the DASH Diet is to avoid sugar and refined carbohydrates and stick with complex carbohydrates. It is one of the top recommended diets for those looking for an alternative lifestyle.

Better Blood Pressure Readings

The DASH diet emphases lowering your blood pressure, which is one of the main medical benefits of this diet. This in turn reduces stress levels, and you end up having more energy throughout the day. This means you will not feel lethargic after meals due to blood sugar crashes. The key to weight loss with the DASH Diet is to avoid sugar and refined carbohydrates and stick with complex carbohydrates. It is one of the top recommended diets for those looking for an alternative lifestyle.

More Energy

The DASH diet focuses on lowering your blood pressure, which is one of the main medical benefits of this diet. This in turn reduces stress levels, and you end up having more energy throughout the day. This means you will not feel lethargic after meals due to blood sugar crashes. The key to weight loss with the DASH Diet is to avoid sugar and refined carbohydrates and stick with complex carbohydrates. It is one of my top recommended diets for those looking for an alternative lifestyle.

BREAKFAST

1

SCALLIONS OMELETTE

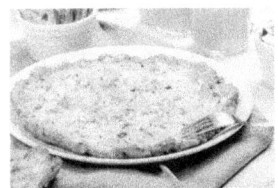

Preparation Time: 10 Minutes
Cooking Time: 10 Minutes
Servings 2
Ingredients
- 1 oz scallions, chopped
- 2 eggs, beaten
- 1 tablespoon low-fat sour cream
- ¼ teaspoon ground black pepper
- 1 teaspoon olive oil

Preparation
1. Heat up olive oil in the skillet.
2. Meanwhile, mix all remaining ingredients into a bowl.
3. Transfer the egg mixture to the hot skillet, flatten well and cook for 7 minutes over medium-low heat.
4. Once set, the omelette is cooked.

Nutritional info
Calories: 101, protein: 6g, carbohydrates: 1.8g, fat: 8g, fibre: 0.4g, cholesterol: 166mg, sodium: 67mg.

2

OVERNIGHT REFRIGERATED OATMEAL

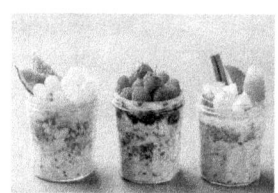

Preparation Time: 5 Minutes
Cooking Time: 5 Minutes
Servings: 1
Ingredients:
- ¼ cup Apples (diced)
- ¼ cup Greek plain yogurt (low-fat)
- ¼ cup Rolled oats
- ¼ cup Applesauce (unsweetened)
- 1/3 cup Soy milk
- 1 ½ teaspoon dried Chia seeds
- ¼ teaspoon Cinnamon

Preparation

1. Add in the soy milk, unsweetened applesauce, rolled oats, low-fat Greek yogurt, diced apples, dried chia seeds, and cinnamon into a 500 ml glass cup with a lid.
2. Close the lid and shake until they are nicely combined.
3. Place the glass cup into the refrigerator overnight.
4. Serve with fresh fruit toppings of your choice.

Nutrition Info

Carbohydrates; 30 g, Sodium; 89 mg, Fat; 4 g, Protein; 11 g

3
APPLE PORRIDGE

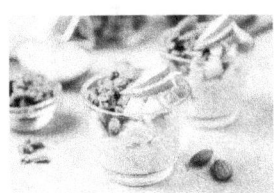

Preparation time: 10 minutes
Cooking time: 4 minutes
Serves: 4
Ingredients
- 2 C. unsweetened almond milk
- 3 tbsp. sunflower seeds
- ½ tsp. organic vanilla extract
- ½ of a small apple, cored and sliced
- 4 tbsp. unsalted walnuts, chopped and divided
- 2 large apples, peeled, cored, and grated
- Pinch of ground cinnamon

Preparation
1. In a large pan, add milk, 2 tbsp. of walnuts, sunflower seeds, grated apple, vanilla, and cinnamon and mix well.
2. Cook on medium-low heat for about 3-4 minutes, stirring occasionally.
3. After cooking, remove from the heat and divide the mixture into 4 serving cups.
4. Top with remaining walnuts and apple slices and serve.

Nutritional Info
Calories: 155, Fat: 7.6g, Carbohydrates: 21.6g, Fibre: 4.6g, Sugar: 14.7g, Protein: 3.2g, Sodium: 92mg

4

HEALTHY BUCKWHEAT PANCAKES

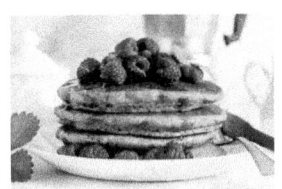

Preparation Time: 10 Minutes
Cooking Time: 30 Minutes
Serving Size: 2
Ingredients:
- ½ cup Buckwheat flour
- 3 cups Fresh sliced strawberries
- 1 tablespoon Canola oil
- ½ cup Milk (fat-free)
- ½ cup All-purpose flour
- 1 tablespoon Sugar
- 2 Egg whites
- ½ cup Sparkling water
- 1 tablespoon Baking powder

Preparation

1. Add the egg whites, milk, and canola oil into a small glass mixing container and whisk until all ingredients are well combined.

2. In another mixing container, add in the all-purpose flour, buckwheat flour, sugar, and baking powder, and whisk together.

3. Add in the egg whites and water. Then whisk into a smooth batter-like consistency and set aside.

4. Take a non-stick griddle and place it over an average flame.

5. Grease it with non-stick cooking spray and let it heat through.

Nutrition Info

Carbohydrates: 24 g, Sodium: 150 mg, Fat: 3 g, Protein: 5 g

5

BANANA BREAD

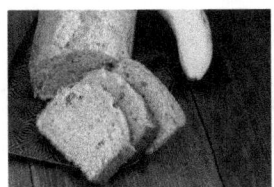

Preparation Time: 10 Minutes
Cooking Time: 1 Hour
Serves: 12
Ingredients
- 1½ C. whole-wheat flour
- ½ C. unsalted walnuts, chopped
- 2 eggs
- 2 tsp. organic vanilla extract
- ¼ C. canola oil
- 1 tsp. powdered stevia
- 1 Pinch of salt
- 1/3 C. fat-free milk
- 1 C. ripe banana, peeled and mashed
- ¼ tsp. ground cardamom

Preparation

1. Preheat the oven to 350 °F. Grease a 9x5-inch loaf pan.

2. In a large container, mix in flour, baking soda, stevia, cardamom, and salt.

3. In another container, add eggs, banana, milk, oil, and vanilla extract and whisk until well combined.

4. Add banana mixture into the flour mixture and mix until just combined. Fold in walnuts.

5. Transfer the mixture into the prepared loaf pan and bake for about an hour.

6. Remove from the oven and put them on a wire rack to cool for 10 minutes. Also, Overturn the bread to cool on the wire rack before cutting.

7. Cut the bread into preferred sized slices and serve.

Nutritional info

Calories: 155, Sodium: 14mg, Carbohydrates: 15.8g, Protein: 4.1g, Fibre: 1.1g, Sugar: 2.1g, Fat: 8.5g

6
ASPARAGUS OMELETTE

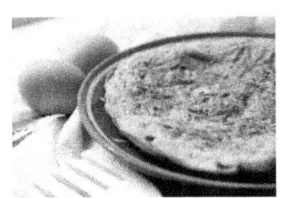

Preparation Time: 5 Minutes
Cooking Time: 10 Minutes
Servings: 2
Ingredients
- 1 teaspoon avocado oil
- ¼ teaspoon ground paprika
- 2 tablespoons low-fat milk
- ½ teaspoon ground cumin
- 3 oz chopped asparagus, boiled
- 3 eggs, beaten

Preparation
1. Heat up avocado oil in the skillet.
2. Meanwhile, mix together ground paprika, ground cumin, eggs, and milk.
3. Pour the liquid into the hot skillet and cook it for 2 minutes.
4. Then add sliced asparagus and close the lid.
5. Cook the omelette for 5 minutes on low heat.

Nutritional Info
Calories: 115, protein: 9.9g, carbohydrates: 3.4g, fat: 7.2g, fibre: 1.2g, sodium: 101mg

7

MUSHROOM SPINACH FRITTATA

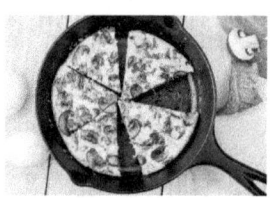

Preparation time: 15 minutes
Cooking time: 40 minutes
Serving size: 6
Ingredients:
- ½ pound sliced Mushrooms
- ¼ cup Feta cheese
- 3 cloves minced Garlic
- 1 teaspoon Dried dill
- 1 cup chopped Onion
- ¼ teaspoon Black pepper
- 10 ounces Fresh spinach
- 1 tablespoon Water
- 10 eggs equivalent Egg substitute
- 1 teaspoon Olive oil
- ½ teaspoon Dried thyme

Preparation
1. Preheat the oven to 350 degrees Fahrenheit.
2. Place a cast-iron skillet over a medium flame. Pour in the olive oil and heat.

3. Add in the onion, garlic, and sauté for around 5 minutes. Toss in the mushrooms and sauté for another 5 minutes.

4. After cooking, remove it from the flame and set it aside.

Nutrition Info

Carbohydrates: 8 g, Fat: 2 g, Protein: 14 g, Sodium: 290 mg

8
EGGS ON TOAST

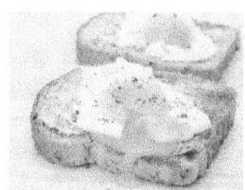

Preparation Time: 10 Minutes
Cooking Time: 3 Minutes
Servings: 2
Ingredients
- 2 whole-wheat bread slices
- 2 large eggs
- 2 tsp. low-fat Parmesan cheese, grated
- Freshly ground black pepper, to taste

Preparation

1. Create a hole at the centre of the bread slice each with a biscuit cutter.
2. Heat a greased non-stick skillet over medium-low heat.
3. Arrange a bread slice in the skillet and carefully crack the egg in the centre of the hole.
4. Cook for about 30-45 seconds. Sprinkle with black pepper and carefully flip the slice. Cook for about 1 minute or until the desired doneness of egg yolk.
5. Repeat with the remaining slice and egg. Sprinkle with parmesan and serve.

Nutritional Info

Calories: 138, Carbohydrates: 10.8g, Sodium: 155mg, Fibre: 1.7g, Fat: 6.1g, Protein: 9.9g

9
SWEET YOGURT WITH FIGS

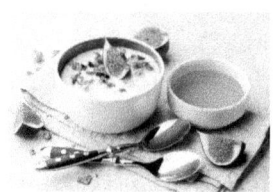

Preparation time: 5 minutes
Cooking time: 0 minutes
1 serving
Ingredients
- 1/3 cup low-fat yogurt
- ¼ teaspoon sesame seeds
- 1 fresh fig, chopped
- 1 teaspoon almond flakes
- 1 teaspoon liquid honey

Preparation

1. Mix together yogurt and honey. Pour the mixture into the serving glass.
2. Top it with sliced fig, almond flakes, and sesame seeds.

Nutritional info

Calories: 178, protein: 6.2g, carbohydrates: 24.4g, fat: 6.8g, fibre: 3.1g, sodium: 44mg

10

GREEN SMOOTHIE

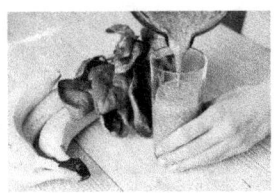

Preparation Time: 2 Minutes
Cooking Time: 5 Minutes
Servings 4
Ingredients
- 2 ounces fresh Baby spinach
- 1 Banana
- 1 cup Cold water
- Fresh mint to taste
- ½ cup Strawberries
- ½ cup Blueberries or blackberries
- 4 tablespoons Lemon juice

Preparation

1. Add in the banana, lemon juice, strawberries, blueberries or blackberries, baby spinach, fresh mint, and cold water into a blender and.
2. Blend into a smooth puree-like consistency.
3. Transfer into a tall glass and serve cold!

Nutrition Info
Protein: 1 g, Carbohydrates: 12 g, Sodium: 5 mg, Fat: 0 g

11

QUINOA BREAD

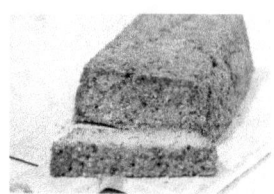

Preparation Time: 15 Minutes
Cooking Time: 1 Hour
Servings: 10
Ingredients
- 2 C. rinsed uncooked quinoa,
- 3 tbsp. unsalted margarine, melted
- ¼ tsp. ground cinnamon
- 2 C. unsweetened almond milk
- 1 tsp. baking soda
- 1 tbsp. black sesame seeds
- 1 C. oat flour
- 1 tsp. organic baking powder
- Pinch of salt
- 1 tbsp. fresh lemon juice

Preparation

1. Preheat the oven to 400 °F. Grease an 8x5-inch loaf pan.

2. In a food processor, add quinoa and pulse until a flour-like texture forms.

3. Transfer the quinoa flour into a large container. Add oat flour, baking soda, baking powder, cinnamon, and salt mix well.

4. In another container, add milk, margarine, and lemon juice and beat until well combined. Add the milk mixture into the flour mixture and mix until well combined.

5. Place the mixture onto the prepared loaf pan evenly and sprinkle with sesame seeds evenly. Cover the loaf pan loosely with a piece of foil.

6. Bake for about 30 minutes. Remove the piece of foil and bake for about 30 minutes more.

7. Remove the loaf pan from the oven and place it onto a wire rack to cool for about 10 minutes.

8. Invert the bread onto the wire rack to cool before slicing.

9. Cut the bread into desired sized slices and serve.

Nutritional Info

Calories: 206, Carbohydrates: 29.1g, Fibre: 3.6g, Protein: 6.4g, Sodium: 200mg, Fat: 7.3g

12
ARTICHOKE EGGS

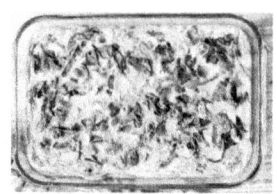

Preparation Time: 5 Minutes
Cook Time: 20 Minutes
Servings 4
Ingredients
- 5 eggs, beaten
- 1 cup artichoke hearts, canned, chopped
- 1 tablespoon cilantro, chopped
- 1 yellow onion, chopped
- 2 oz low-fat feta, chopped
- 1 tablespoon canola oil

Preparation
1. Grease 4 ramekins with oil.
2. Mix up all remaining ingredients and divide the mixture between prepared ramekins.
3. Bake the meal at 380F for 20 minutes.

Nutrition Info
Calories: 177, protein: 10.6, carbohydrates: 7.4g, fat: 12.2g, fibre: 2.5g, sodium: 259mg.

13
MUESLI BARS

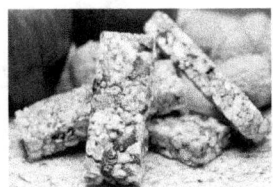

Preparation time: 10 minutes
Cooking Time: 15 Minutes
Servings: 8
Ingredients:
- 2 ½ cups Rolled oats (old-fashioned)
- 1 cup Dark honey
- ½ cup Soy flour
- ½ cup toasted Wheat germ
- 2 teaspoons Vanilla extract
- 1 tablespoon Olive oil
- ½ cup chopped Dried apples
- ½ cup Raisins
- ½ cup Dry milk (fat-free)
- ½ cup sliced Toasted almonds
- ½ cup unsalted Natural peanut butter
- ½ teaspoon Salt

Preparation
1. Begin by preheating the oven by setting the temperature to 325 degrees Fahrenheit.

2. Take a 9x13 baking dish and grease it with non-stick cooking spray. Set it aside

3. In a large glass bowl, add in the flour, oats, dry milk, almonds, wheat germ, apples, salt, and raisins. Mix well and set aside.

4. Take a small saucepan and place it on a medium-low flame. Pour in the olive oil and let it get warm.

5. Add in the peanut butter and honey and mix until it is well combined; let it come to a boil.

6. Once the mixture boils, stir in the vanilla. Remove from the flame.

7. Pour the prepared honey mixture into the flour and oats mixture. Mix quickly until the ingredients are perfectly combined. Make sure there are no lumps at all.

8. Transfer the mixture to the greased baking dish and press to get rid of any air pockets.

9. Place the baking dish into the preheated oven and bake for around 25 minutes.

10. Once done, take the dish out of the oven, and place it on a wire rack. Allow it to rest for about 10 minutes.

11. Use a sharp knife to cut 24 equal-sized bars. Remove them carefully once cut. Place the bars on the wire rack until they are completely cooled.

12. store the bars in the fridge in an airtight glass container.

Nutritional Info

Protein: 5 g, Sodium: 81 mg, Carbohydrates; 26 g Fat; 5 g

14

SWEET POTATO TOAST

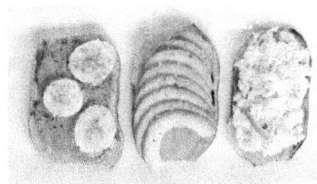

Preparation time: 15 minutes
Cooking time: 25 minutes
Servings:
Ingredients:
- 1 large unpeeled sweet potato

Topping Choice 1
- 1 ripe banana, sliced
- Dash of ground cinnamon
- 4 tablespoons peanut butter

Topping Choice 2:
- 2 eggs (1 per slice)
- ½ mashed avocado

Topping Choice 3:
- 1 sliced tomato
- Dash of black pepper
- 4 tablespoons low-fat ricotta cheese

Preparation
1. Cut the sweet potato into ¼-inch thick slices.
2. Place the sweet potato slices in a toaster and heat on high for about 5 minutes or until cooked through.

3. Repeat multiple times, if necessary, depending on the toaster settings.

4. Top with your desired topping choices and enjoy.

Nutritional Info

Calories: 137, Carbohydrates: 32g, Sodium: 17mg, Fibre: 4g, Protein: 2g, Fat: 0g

15

CINNAMON AND COCONUT PORRIDGE

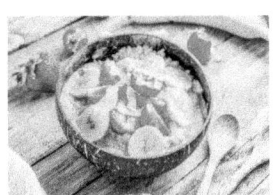

Prep Time: 5 minutes
Cook Time: 5 minutes
Serving: 4
Ingredients:
- ½ teaspoon cinnamon
- 1/2 tablespoon almond butter
- 1/2 cup 36-percent low-fat cream
- 1 ½ teaspoons stevia
- 1 tablespoon flaxseed meal
- 1 tablespoon oat bran
- 1 cup water
- ½ cup unsweetened dried coconut, shredded
- Toppings, such as blueberries or banana slices, etc

Preparation

1. Add the ingredients to a small pot and mix well until fully combined
2. Transfer over medium-low heat and bring the mix to a slow boil.
3. Stir well and remove from the heat.

4.Divide the mixture into equal servings and let them sit for 10 minutes.

5.Top with your preferred toppings and enjoy!

Nutritional info

Calories: 171, Carbohydrates: 8g, Protein: 2g, Fat: 16g

16

BAKING POWDER BISCUITS

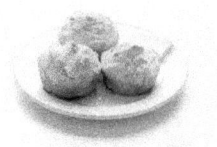

Preparation Time: 5 Minutes
Cooking Time: 5 Minutes
Servings: 1
Ingredients:
- 1 c. all-purpose flour
- 2/3 c. low-Fat milk
- 1 egg white
- 4 tbsps. vegetable shortening (Non-hydrogenated)
- 1 tbsp. sugar
- 1 c. white whole-wheat flour
- 4 tsp. Sodium-free baking powder

Preparation

1. Warm oven to 450°F. Put the flour, sugar, plus baking powder into a mixing container and mix.

2. Split the shortening into the batter using your fingers until it looks like coarse crumbs. Add in the egg white, milk, and stir to combine.

3. On a lightly floured surface Place and knead the dough for a minute. Roll into ¾ inch thick and cut into 12 rounds.

4.Place the rounds on the baking sheet and bake for 10 minutes. then

5.After baking, remove the baking sheet and place biscuits on a wire rack to cool.

Nutritional info

Calories: 118, Carbohydrates:16 g, Protein:3 g, Fat:4 g, Sugars:0.2 g, Sodium: 6 mg

17
ALMOND BUTTER BANANA CHOCOLATE SMOOTHIE

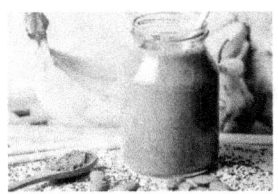

Preparation Time: 5 Minutes
Servings: 1
Ingredients
- ½ medium banana, preferably frozen
- 1 tablespoon unsweetened cocoa powder
- 1 tablespoon chia seeds
- 1 tablespoon almond butter
- ¾ cup almond milk
- ¼ cup frozen blueberries

Preparation
Add and pulse all ingredients in a blender until it combines.
Nutritional Info
Calories: 300 fat: 16g; Sodium: 125mg; Carbohydrates: 37g; Fibre: 10g; Sugars: 17g; Protein: 8g

18

AVOCADO TOAST WITH SMOKED TROUT

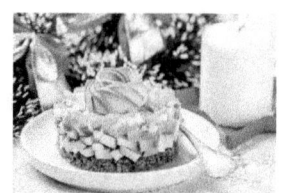

Preparation Time: 10 Minutes
Servings 2
Ingredients
- 1 peeled and pitted avocado,
- 4-ounce smoked trout
- ¼ teaspoon kosher salt
- ¼ teaspoon lemon zest
- 2 pieces whole-wheat bread, toasted
- ¾ teaspoon ground cumin
- 2 teaspoons lemon juice, plus more for serving
- ¼ teaspoon red pepper flakes

Preparation

1. In a medium container, mash together the avocado, lemon juice, cumin, salt, red pepper flakes, and lemon zest.

2. On each toast piece, spread half of the mixture. Top each of the toasted pieces with half the smoked trout.

3. If desire, garnish with a pinch of red pepper flakes and a sprinkle of lemon juice.

Nutritional Info

Calories: 300; fat: 20g; Sodium: 390mg; Carbohydrates: 21g; Fibre: 6g; Sugars: 1g; Protein: 11g

19

CRUNCHY FLAX AND ALMOND CRACKERS

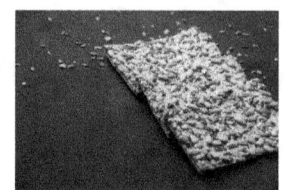

Preparation Time: 15 Minutes
Cooking Time: 60 Minutes
Servings: 24 Crackers
Ingredients:
- ½ cup ground flaxseeds
- ½ cup almond flour
- 1 tablespoon coconut flour
- 1 egg white
- ¼ teaspoon sunflower seeds
- 2 tablespoons shelled hemp seeds
- 2 tablespoons unsalted almond butter, melted

Preparation
1. Preheat your oven to 300 degrees F.
2. Hold a baking sheet lined with parchment paper to the side.
3. Add flax, almond, coconut flour, hemp seed, seeds to a bowl and mix.
4. Add egg white and melted almond butter, mix until combined.
5. Transfer dough to a sheet of parchment paper and cover with another sheet of paper.

6. Roll out dough and cut into crackers
7. Bake for 60 minutes. Let them cool and enjoy!

Nutritional Info

Calories 173, Carbohydrates: 1.2 g, Protein: 2g, Fat: 6g, Fibre: 1g

20

GRAPE YOGURT

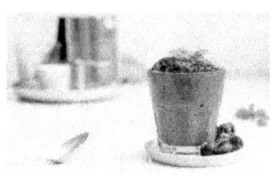

Prep time: 10 minutes

Cook time: 0 minutes

servings 3

Ingredients

- ½ cup chopped grapes
- 1 ½ cup low-fat yogurt
- 1 oz chopped walnuts

Preparation

Mix up all ingredients together and transfer them to the serving glasses.

Nutritional info

Calories: 156, protein: 9.4g, carbohydrates; 12.2g, fat: 7.1g, fibre: 0.8g, sodium: 86mg

LUNCH

21

STIR-FRY RICE WITH CHICKEN

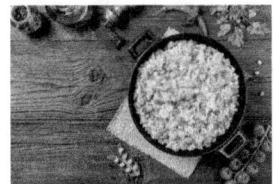

Preparation Time: 10 Minutes
Cooking Time: 30 Minutes
Servings: 4
Ingredients:
- 1/3 cup rice wine vinegar
- 2 tablespoons olive oil
- ½ cup coconut aminos
- 1 lb chicken breast dice into 1-inch cube
- ½ cup chopped red bell pepper,
- A pinch of black pepper
- ½ teaspoon ginger, grated
- ½ cup carrots, grated 1 cup white rice
- 2 garlic cloves, minced

Preparation

1. Heat-up a pan with the oil over medium-high heat, add the chicken and stir for 4 minutes on each side.

2. Add aminos, vinegar, bell pepper, black pepper, garlic, ginger, carrots, rice, and stock. Cover the pan and cook over medium-heat for 20 minutes.

3.Divide everything into bowls and serve for lunch. Enjoy!
Nutritional Info
Calories: 70, Carbohydrates: 13g, Fat: 2g, Protein: 2g, Sodium 5 mg

22

SPINACH AND BEEF MEATBALLS

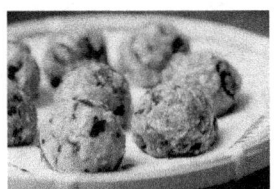

Prep Time: 10 minutes

Cooking Time: 20

Servings: 4

Ingredients:
- 10 ounces spinach
- Pepper as needed
- 1 whole egg
- ½ cup onion
- ¼ teaspoon oregano
- 1-pound lean ground beef
- 4 garlic cloves

Preparation

1. Preheat your oven to 375 degrees F.
2. In a bowl, mix in the rest of the ingredients using your hands, and roll into meatballs.
3. Transfer to a sheet tray and bake for 20 minutes.
4. Once done, serve and enjoy!

Nutritional Info

Calorie: 200, Fat: 8g, Carbohydrates: 5g, Protein: 29g

23
FAUX MAC AND CHEESE

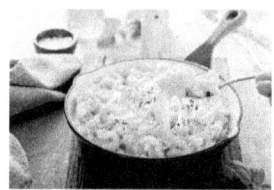

Preparation Time: 15 minutes
Cooking Time: 45 minutes
Serving: 4
Ingredients
- 5 cups cauliflower florets
- 1 cup cashew cheese
- Sunflower seeds and pepper to taste
- ½ cup vegetable broth
- 1 organic egg, beaten
- 1 cup coconut almond milk
- 2 tablespoons coconut flour, sifted

Preparation
1. Preheat your oven to 350 degrees F.
2. Season florets with sunflower seeds and steam until firm.
3. Place florets in a greased ovenproof dish.
4. Heat coconut almond milk over medium heat in a skillet, make sure to season the oil with sunflower seeds and pepper.
5. Stir in broth and add coconut flour to the mix, stir.
6. Cook until the sauce begins to bubble.
7. Remove heat and add beaten egg.

8. Pour the thick sauce over the cauliflower and mix in cheese.
9. Bake for 35 minutes.
10. Serve and enjoy!

Nutritional Info

Calories: 229, Protein: 15g, Fat: 14g, Carbohydrates: 9g

24

PURPLE POTATO SOUP

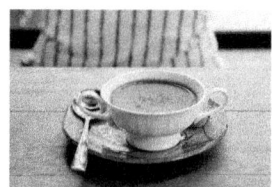

Preparation time: 10 minutes
Cooking time: 1 hour and 15 minutes
Servings: 6
Ingredients:
- 6 chopped purple potatoes
- 1 cauliflower head, florets separated
- Black pepper to the taste
- 4 garlic cloves, minced
- 1 yellow onion, chopped
- 3 tablespoons olive oil
- tablespoon thyme, chopped
- 1 chopped leek
- Chopped shallots
- 4 cups chicken stock, low-sodium

Preparation

1. In a baking dish, mix potatoes with onion, cauliflower, garlic, pepper, thyme, and half of the oil,

2. Toss to coat, introduce in the oven and bake for 45 minutes at 400 degrees F.

3. Heat the pot with the rest of the oil over medium-high heat, add leeks and shallots, stir and cook for 10 minutes.

4. Add roasted veggies and stock, stir, cook for 20 minutes.

5. Transfer soup to your food processor, blend well, divide into bowls, and serve.

Nutritional Info

Calories: 70 Carbohydrates: 15g Fat: 0g Protein: 2g Sodium 6 mg

25

TURKEY LETTUCE WRAP

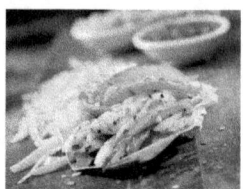

Preparation Time: 10 minutes
Cooking Time: 10 minutes
Servings: 6
Ingredients:
- 1 ¼ pounds ground turkey, lean
- 12 almond butter lettuce leaves
- 1 tablespoon olive oil
- 2 teaspoons chili paste
- 1 garlic clove, minced
- 4 green onions, minced
- 3 tablespoons hoisin sauce
- 1 tablespoon rice vinegar
- 1/8 teaspoon sunflower seeds
- 2 tablespoon coconut aminos
- 8-ounce water chestnut, diced

Preparation

1. Place a pan over medium heat, add turkey, oil, and garlic to the pan.
2. Heat for 6 minutes until cooked.
3. Transfer turkey to a container.

4. Add onions and water chestnuts.
5. Stir in hoisin sauce, coconut aminos, vinegar, and chili paste.
6. Toss well and transfer the mix to lettuce leaves.
7. Serve and enjoy!

Nutritional Info

Calories: 162, Carbohydrates: 7g, Protein: 23g, Fat: 4g

26

EASY SALMON STEAKS

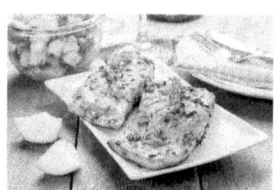

Preparation time: 10 minutes
Cooking time: 20 minutes
Servings: 4
Ingredients:
- 1 big salmon fillet, cut into 4 steaks
- 2 tablespoons olive oil
- 1 tablespoon thyme, chopped
- Black pepper to the taste
- 4 cups of water
- ¼ cup parsley, chopped
- 1 lemon Juice
- 1 yellow onion, chopped
- 3 garlic cloves, minced

Preparation

1. Place a pan with the oil on medium-high heat, cook onion and garlic within 3 minutes.

2. Add black pepper, parsley, thyme, water, and lemon juice, stir, bring to a gentle boil.

3. Add salmon steaks, cook them for 15 minutes, drain, divide between plates and serve with a side salad for lunch.

Nutritional Info

Calories: 110, Carbohydrates: 3g, Fat: 4g, Protein: 15g, Sodium 330 mg

27

CHICKEN AND CARROT STEW

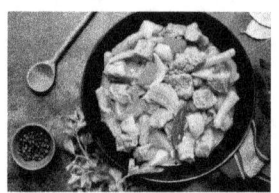

Preparation Time: 15 minutes
Cooking Time: 6 hours
Servings: 4
Ingredients:
- 2 cups of chicken broth
- 4 boneless chicken breasts, cubed
- 1 cup onion, chopped
- 3 cups of carrots, peeled and cubed
- 1 teaspoon of dried thyme
- 2 garlic cloves, minced
- 1 cup tomatoes, chopped

Preparation
1. Add all of the itemised ingredients to a Slow Cooker.
2. Stir and close the lid.
3. Cook for 6 hours.
4. Serve hot and enjoy!

Nutritional Info
Calories: 182, Fat: 3g, Protein: 39g, Carbohydrates: 10g

28

LEEKS SOUP

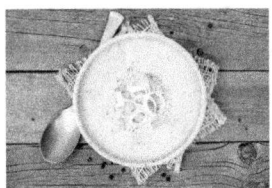

Preparation Time: 10 Minutes
Cooking Time: 1 Hour And 15 Minutes
Servings: 6
Ingredients:
- 2 gold potatoes, chopped
- 1 cup cauliflower florets
- Black pepper to the taste
- 5 leeks, chopped
- garlic cloves, minced
- 1 yellow onion, chopped
- 3 tablespoons olive oil
- Handful parsley, chopped
- 4 cups low-sodium chicken stock

Preparation

1. Heat-up a pot with the oil over medium-high heat, add onion and garlic, stir and cook for 5 minutes.

2. Add potatoes, cauliflower, black pepper, leeks, and stock, stir, bring to a simmer, cook over medium heat for 30 minutes

3. Blend using an immersion blender, add parsley, stir, ladle into bowls and serve.

Nutritional Info

Calories: 125 carbohydrates: 29g Fat: 1g Protein: 4g Sodium 52 mg

29
PISTACHIO MINT PESTO PASTA

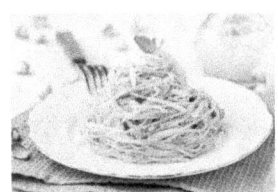

Preparation Time: 10 Minutes
Cooking Time: 10 Minutes
Servings 4
Ingredients
- 8 ounces whole-wheat pasta
- ⅓ cup extra-virgin olive oil
- ⅓ cup unsalted pistachios, shelled
- 1 cup fresh mint
- ½ cup fresh basil
- 1 garlic clove, peeled
- Juice of ½ lime
- ½ teaspoon kosher salt

Preparation

1. Prepare the pasta based on the package instructions. Drain, reserving ½ cup of the pasta water, and set aside.

2. In a food processor, add the mint, basil, pistachios, garlic, salt, and lime juice. Process until the pistachios are coarsely ground. Add the olive oil in a slow, steady stream and process until combined.

3. In a large container, mix the pasta with the pistachio pesto; toss well to combine.

4. If using a thinner, more saucy consistency is desired, add some of the reserved pasta water and toss well.

Nutritional Info

Calories: 420; fat: 3g; Sodium: 150mg; Carbohydrates: 48g; Fibre: 2g; Protein: 11g;

30

LAMB CURRY WITH TOMATOES AND SPINACH

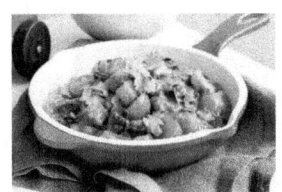

Preparation Time: 10 Minutes
Cooking Time: 12 Minutes
Servings: 4
Ingredients
- 2 Tbsp. Salt-free tomato paste
- 1 tsp. Olive oil
- 1, chopped Onion
- 3 cloves, minced Garlic
- Ground black pepper to taste
- 1, chopped Red bell pepper
- 1 Tbsp. Salt-free curry powder
- ¼ cup Chopped fresh cilantro
- 1 pound sliced thinly Lean boneless lamb
- 10 ounces Fresh baby spinach
- ½ cup Low-sodium beef or vegetable broth
- ¼ cup Red wine
- 1(15-ounce) can No-salt-added diced tomatoes

Preparation
1. Heat the oil in a pan.
2. Add lamb and brown on both sides, about 2 minutes.

3. Add garlic, onion, and bell pepper. Stir-fry for 2 minutes. Add in and Stir the curry powder and tomato paste.

4. Add the tomatoes with juice, spinach, broth, and wine and stir to mix.

5. Stir-fry for 3 to 4 minutes and lamb has cooked through.

6. Remove from heat. Season with pepper and stir in cilantro. Serve.

Nutritional Info

Calories: 238, Sodium 167mg, Fat: 7g, carbohydrates: 14g, Protein: 27g

31

ZUCCHINI ZOODLES WITH CHICKEN AND BASIL

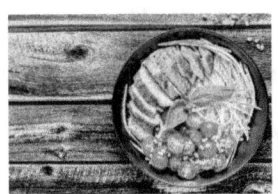

Preparation Time: 10 minutes
Cooking Time: 10 minutes
Serving: 3
Ingredients:
- 1 zucchini, shredded
- 2 tablespoons ghee
- 1 garlic clove, peeled, minced
- 2 chicken fillets, cubed
- ½ cup basil, chopped
- ¼ cup almond milk
- 1-pound tomatoes, diced

Preparation
1. Sauté cubed chicken in ghee until no longer pink.
2. Add tomatoes and season with sunflower seeds.
3. Simmer and reduce the liquid.
4. Prepare your zucchini Zoodles by shredding zucchini in a food processor.
5. Add basil, garlic, coconut almond milk to the chicken and cook for a few minutes.

6.Add half of the zucchini Zoodles to a bowl and top with creamy tomato basil chicken. Enjoy!

Nutritional Info

Calories: 540, Carbohydrates: 13g, Fat: 27g, Protein: 59g

32

INDIAN CHICKEN STEW

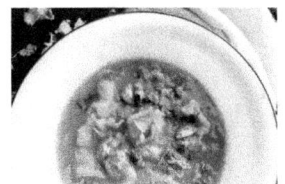

Preparation time: 55 minutes
Cooking time: 20 minutes
Servings: 4
Ingredients:
- 1-pound chicken breasts, skinless, boneless, and cubed
- 15 ounces tomato sauce,
- 5 garlic cloves, minced
- ½ teaspoon sweet paprika
- 1 tablespoon garam masala
- 1 tablespoon lemon juice
- A pinch of black pepper
- ¼ teaspoon ginger, ground
- 1 cup fat-free yogurt

Preparation

1. In a bowl, mix the chicken with garam masala, yogurt, lemon juice, black pepper, ginger, and fridge for 1 hour.

2. Heat-up a pan over medium heat, add chicken mix, toss and cook for 5-6 minutes.

3. Add tomato sauce, garlic and paprika, toss, cook for 15 minutes, divide between plates and serve

Nutritional Info
Calories 221, Fat 6g, Fibre 9g, carbohydrates 14g, Sodium 4 mg, Protein 16g

33

GOLDEN EGGPLANT FRIES

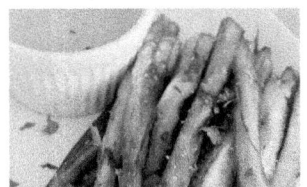

Preparation Time: 10 minutes

Cooking Time: 15 minutes

Serving: 8

Ingredients:

- 2 eggplant, peeled and cut thinly
- 2 eggs
- 2 cups almond flour
- 2 tablespoons coconut oil, spray
- Sunflower seeds and pepper

Preparation

1. Preheat your oven to 400 degrees F.
2. In a container, add and mix sunflower seeds and black pepper.
3. In another container and beat eggs until frothy.
4. Dip the eggplant pieces into the eggs.
5. Then coat them with the flour mixture.
6. Add another layer of flour and egg.
7. Then, take a baking sheet and grease with coconut oil on top.

8.Bake for about 15 minutes. Serve and enjoy!
Nutritional info
Calories: 212 Fat: 15.8g Protein: 8.6g Carbohydrates: 12.1g

34

CAULIFLOWER LUNCH SALAD

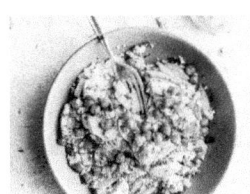

Preparation time: 10 minutes
Cooking time: 10 minutes
Servings: 4
Ingredients:
- 1/3 cup low-sodium veggie stock
- 2 tablespoons olive oil
- 6 cups cauliflower florets, grated
- Black pepper to the taste
- 1/4 cup red onion, chopped
- 1 red bell pepper, chopped
- Juice of 1/2 lemon
- 2 cup kalamata olives halved
- 1 teaspoon mint, chopped
- 1 tablespoon cilantro, chopped

Preparation

1. Heat-up a pan with the oil over medium-high heat, add cauliflower, pepper, and stock, stir, cook within 10 minutes
2. Transfer to a container, and keep in the fridge for 2 hours.
3. Mix cauliflower with olives, onion, bell pepper, black pepper, mint, cilantro, and lemon juice, toss to coat and serve.

Nutritional info:

Calories: 102, Sodium 97 mg, carbohydrates: 3g, Fat: 10g, Protein: 0g

35

TROUT PARCEL

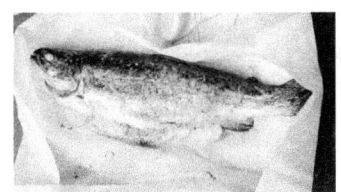

Preparation time: 10 minutes
Cooking time: 20 minutes
Servings: 2
Ingredients
- 2 (4-oz.) rainbow trout fillets
- 1 jalapeño pepper, sliced
- 1 lemon, sliced
- 1 tbsp. olive oil
- Pinch of salt
- Freshly ground black pepper, to taste

Preparation

1. Preheat the oven to 400 °F. In a container, add trout fillets, garlic salt, black pepper, and oil and toss to coat well.

2. Arrange both fillets onto a large piece of foil. Divide jalapeño slices over both fillets evenly.

3. Drizzle with some lemon juice. Top with 1-2 lemon slices. Cover the trout fillets by sealing all edges to form a parcel.

4. Arrange the foil parcels into a baking sheet in a single layer. Bake for about 15-20 minutes.

5. Remove from oven and place parcels onto a platter. Carefully open each parcel and serve.

Nutritional Info

Calories: 280 Fat: 16.7g Sodium: 144mg Fibre: 0.4g Sugar: 0.4g carbohydrates: 1.1g Protein: 30.4g

36

SPINACH PORK CUBES

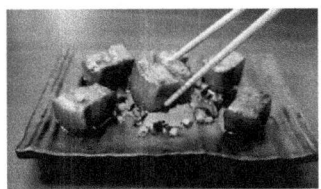

Preparation Time: 10 Minutes
Cooking Time: 12 Minutes
Servings: 4
Ingredients
- 4 pork loin chops, cubed
- 4 teaspoons spinach, blended

Preparation
1. Mix up pork chops and blended spinach.
2. Then preheat the grill to 400F.
3. Put the meat cubes in the grill and roast them for 6 minutes per side or until the meat is light brown.
4. Serve.

Nutritional Info
Calories 256, sodium 57mg, protein 18g, carbohydrates 0g, fat 19.9g, fibre 0g

37
TILAPIA CASSEROLE

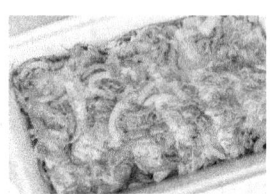

Preparation Time: 10 Minutes
Cooking Time: 14 Minutes
Servings: 4
Ingredients
- 4 (6-oz.) tilapia fillets
- 2 tbsp. fresh lemon juice
- ½ tsp. red pepper flakes, crushed
- 1/3 C. fresh parsley, chopped and divided
- 2/3 C. feta cheese, crumbled
- ¼ tsp. dried oregano
- 2 (14-oz.) cans salt-free diced tomatoes with basil and garlic with juice

Preparation
1. Preheat the oven to 400 °F.
2. Using a shallow baking dish, add in the tomatoes, ¼ C. of the parsley, oregano, and red pepper flakes and mix until well combined.
3. Arrange the tilapia fillets over the tomato mixture in a single layer and drizzle with the lemon juice.
4. Place some tomato mixture over the tilapia fillets and

sprinkle with the feta cheese evenly. Bake for about 12-14 minutes.

5. Serve hot with the garnishing of remaining parsley.

Nutritional Info

Calories: 246, Sodium: 350mg, carbohydrates: 9.4g, Fibre: 2.7g, Fat: 7.4g, Protein: 37.2g, Sugar: 6g

38

BALSAMIC VINEGAR STEAK

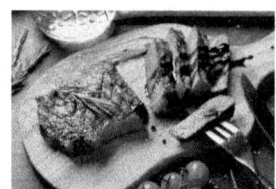

Preparation Time: 20 Minutes

Cooking Time: 20 Minutes

Servings: 2

Ingredients

- 1/3 cup balsamic vinegar
- 1 tablespoon canola oil
- 2 beef sirloin steaks
- 1 teaspoon dried thyme

Preparation

1. Mix up balsamic vinegar and dried thyme.

2. Put the meat in the vinegar mixture and leave it to marinate for 15 minutes.

3. Then preheat the canola oil in the skillet.

4. Add steaks and cook them for 10 minutes per side on medium heat.

5. Slice the cooked beef steaks.

Nutritional Info

Calories 230, protein 25.9g, carbohydrates 0.7g, fat 12.3g, fibre 0.2g, sodium 58mg

39

SHRIMP WITH ASPARAGUS

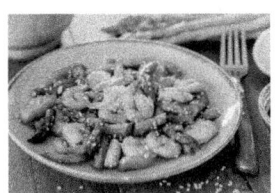

Preparation Time: 15 Minutes
Cooking Time: 10 Minutes
Servings: 4
Ingredients
- 1 lb. shrimp, peeled and deveined
- 2 tbsp. fresh lemon juice
- 1/3 C. low-sodium chicken broth
- 4 garlic cloves, minced
- 2 tbsp. olive oil
- 1 lb. asparagus, trimmed

Preparation

1. In a large frying pan with oil over medium-high heat, apply heat. Add all the ingredients except for broth and cook for about 2 minutes, without stirring.

2. Stir the mixture and cook for about 3-4 minutes, stirring occasionally.

3. Stir in the broth and cook for about 2-4 more minutes. Serve hot.

Nutritional Info

Calories: 225, Fat: 9.1g, Sodium: 280mg, Fibre: 2.5g, Sugar: 2.2g, Protein: 28.7g, Carbohydrates: 7.4g

40

TRADITIONAL BLACK BEAN CHILI

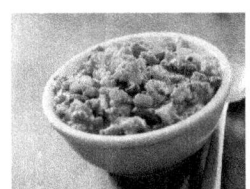

Preparation Time: 10 minutes
Cooking Time: 4 hours
Serving: 4
Ingredients:
- 16 ounces canned black beans
- 1 cup yellow onion, chopped
- 1 ½ cups mushrooms, sliced
- 1 tablespoon chili powder
- ½ teaspoon cumin, ground
- 1 ½ cups red bell pepper, chopped
- 1 cup tomatoes, chopped
- 2 tablespoons cilantro, chopped
- 2 garlic cloves, minced
- 1 teaspoon chipotle chili pepper, chopped
- 1 tablespoon olive oil

Preparation

1. Add red bell peppers, onion, dill, mushrooms, chili powder, garlic, chili pepper, cumin, black beans, tomatoes to your Slow Cooker.

2. Stir well and cover the slow.
3. Cook on HIGH.
4. Sprinkle cilantro on top. Serve and enjoy!

Nutritional Info

Calories: 211, Carbohydrates: 22g, Protein: 5g, Fat: 3g

DINNER

41

PAPRIKA LAMB CHOPS

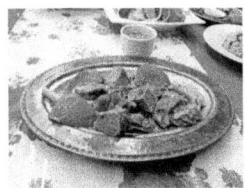

Preparation Time: 10 Minutes
Cooking Time: 15 Minutes
Serving: 4
Ingredients:
- 1 lamb rack, cut into chops
- 1/2 teaspoon chili powder
- 1/2 cup cumin powder
- 1 tablespoon paprika

Preparation
1. In a container, add and stir paprika, cumin, chili, pepper.
2. Add lamb chops and rub the mixture.
3. Heat grill over medium-temperature and add lamb chops, cook for 5 minutes.
4. Turn it over and cook for e5 minutes, flip again.
5. Cook for 2 minutes, flip and cook for 2 minutes more.
6. Serve and enjoy!

Nutritional Info
Calories: 200, Fat: 5g, Carbohydrates 4g, Protein: 8g

42

SHRIMP COCKTAIL

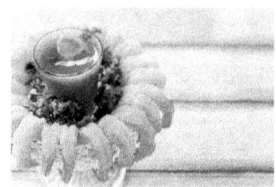

Preparation Time: 10 Minutes
Cooking Time: 5 Minutes
Servings: 8
Ingredients:
- 2 pounds big shrimp, deveined
- 1 medium lemon sliced for serving
- 1 small lemon, halved
- Ice for cooling the shrimp
- 2 tablespoons lemon juice
- 2 and ½ tablespoons horseradish, prepared
- 4 cups of water
- ¾ cup tomato passata
- ¼ teaspoon chili powder
- 2 bay leaves
- Ice for serving

Preparation

1. Pour the 4 cups water into a large pot, add lemon and bay leaves. Boil over medium-high heat, reduce temperature and boil for 10 minutes.

2.Put shrimp, stir and cook within 2 minutes. Move the shrimp to a container filled with ice and leave aside for 5 minutes.

3.In another container, mix tomato passata with horseradish, chili powder, and lemon juice and stir well.

4.Place shrimp in a serving bowl filled with ice, with lemon slices, and serve with the cocktail sauce prepared.

Nutritional Info

Calories: 276, Carbohydrates: 0g, Protein: 25g, Sodium: 182 mg, Fat: 8g

43

BEEF AND ONION STEW

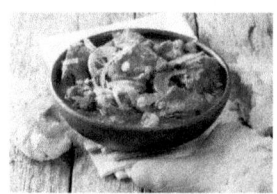

Preparation Time: 10 minutes
Cooking Time 1-2 hours
Servings: 4
Ingredients:
- 2 pounds lean beef, cubed
- ¼ cup olive oil
- 3 tablespoons lemon juice
- 3 tablespoons tomato paste
- 5 garlic cloves, peeled, whole
- 1 bay leaves
- 3 pounds shallots, peeled
- 2 medium carrot, diced

Preparation
1. Take a stew pot and place it over medium heat.
2. Add olive oil and let it heat up.
3. Add meat and brown.
4. Add remaining ingredients and cover with water.
5. Bring the whole mix to a boil.
6. Reduce heat to low and cover the pot.

7.Simmer for 1-2 hours until beef is cooked thoroughly. Serve hot!

Nutritional Info

Calories: 136, Carbohydrates: 0.9g, Protein: 24g, Fat: 3g

44

SHRIMP WITH WHITE BEANS AND FETA

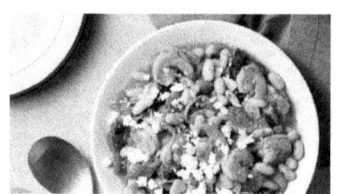

Preparation Time: 15 Minutes
Cooking Time: 15 Minutes
Servings 4
Ingredients
- 3 tablespoons lemon juice, divided
- 2 tablespoons extra-virgin olive oil, divided
- ½ teaspoon kosher salt, divided
- 1 pound shrimp, peeled and deveined
- 1 large shallot, diced
- ¼ cup no-salt-added vegetable stock
- 1 (15-ounce) can no-salt-added or low-sodium cannellini beans, rinsed and drained
- ¼ cup fresh mint, chopped
- 1 teaspoon lemon zest
- 1 tablespoon white wine vinegar
- ¼ teaspoon freshly ground black pepper
- ¼ cup crumbled feta cheese, for garnish

Preparation
1. In a small container, whisk together 1 tablespoon of the

lemon juice, 1 tablespoon of the olive oil, and ¼ teaspoon of the salt. Add the shrimp and set aside.

2. In a large skillet, heat what is left of the olive oil or sauté pan over medium heat.

3. Add the shallot and sauté until translucent, about 2 to 3 minutes. Add the vegetable stock and deglaze the pan, scraping up any brown bits, and bring to a boil.

4. Add the beans and shrimp. Lower the heat, and simmer until shrimp are cooked for about 3 to 4 minutes.

5. Turn off the heat and add the mint, lemon zest, vinegar, and black pepper. Stir gently to combine. Garnish with the feta.

Nutritional Info

Calories: 340; fat: 11g; Sodium: 45mg; Carbohydrates: 28g; Fibre: 6g; Sugars: 3g; Protein: 32g;

45

MUSSELS AND CHICKPEA SOUP

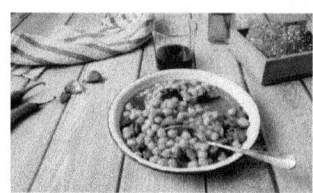

Preparation Time: 10 Minutes
Cooking Time: 10 Minutes
Servings: 6
Ingredients:
- 3 garlic cloves, minced
- 1 and ½ tablespoons fresh mussels, scrubbed
- 3 tablespoons parsley, chopped
- 2 tablespoons olive oil
- 1 small fennel bulb, sliced
- Black pepper to the taste
- 1 cup chickpeas, rinsed
- 1 cup white wine
- Juice of 1 lemon
- A pinch of chili flakes

Preparation

1. Heat a big saucepan with the olive oil over medium-high heat, add garlic and chili flakes, stir and cook within a couple of minutes.

2. Add white wine and mussels, stir, cover, and cook for 3-4 minutes until mussels open.

3. Transfer mussels to a baking dish, add some of the cooking liquid over them and fridge until they are cold enough. Take mussels out of the fridge and discard shells.

4. Heat another pan over medium-high heat, add mussels, reserved cooking liquid, chickpeas, and fennel, stir well, and heat them.

5. Add black pepper to taste, lemon juice, and parsley, stir again, divide between plates and serve.

Nutritional Info

Calories: 286, Carbohydrates: 49g, Fat: 4g, Protein: 14g, Sodium: 145mg

46

WALNUTS AND ASPARAGUS DELIGHT

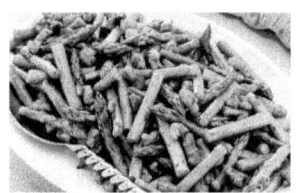

Preparation Time: 5 Minutes
Cooking Time: 5 Minutes
Serving: 4
Ingredients:
- ¾ pound asparagus, trimmed
- Sunflower seeds and pepper to taste
- ¼ cup walnuts, chopped
- 1 ½ tablespoon olive oil

Preparation
1. Over medium heat, place a skillet and add olive oil.
2. Add asparagus, sauté for 5 minutes until browned.
3. Season with sunflower seeds and pepper.
4. Remove heat.
5. Add walnuts and toss. Serve warm!

Nutritional Info
Calories: 124, Protein: 3g, Carbohydrates: 2g, Fat: 12g

QUINOA AND SCALLOPS SALAD

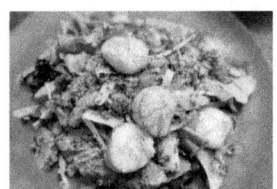

Preparation Time:10 Minutes
Cooking Time:35 Minutes
Servings: 6
Ingredients
- 12 ounces dry sea scallops 4 tablespoons canola oil
- 4 teaspoons low sodium soy sauce
- 2 teaspoons canola oil
- 1 cup snow peas, sliced diagonally 1 teaspoon sesame oil
- ¼ cup cilantro, chopped
- 1/3 cup rice vinegar
- 1 and ½ cup quinoa, rinsed
- 2 teaspoons garlic, minced
- 1 cup scallions, sliced
- 1/3 cup red bell pepper, chopped

Preparation

1. In a bowl, mix scallops with 2 teaspoons soy sauce, stir gently and leave aside for now. Heat a pan with 1 tablespoon canola oil over medium- high heat, add the quinoa, stir and cook for 8 minutes. Put garlic, stir and cook within 1 more minute.

2. Put the water, boil over medium heat, stir, cover, and cook

for 15 minutes. Remove from heat and leave aside covered for 5 minutes. Add snow peas, cover again and leave for 5 more minutes.

3.Meanwhile, in a bowl, mix 3 tablespoons of canola oil with 2 teaspoons soy sauce, vinegar, and sesame oil and stir well. Add quinoa and snow peas to this mixture and stir again. Add scallions, bell pepper, and stir again.

4.Pat dries the scallops and discard marinade. Heat another pan with 2 teaspoons canola oil over high heat, add scallops, and cook for 1 minute on each side. Add them to the quinoa salad, stir gently, and serve with chopped cilantro.

Nutritional Info

Calories: 181, Carbohydrates: 12g, Fat: 6g, Protein: 13g, Sodium: 153 mg

48

FISH STEW

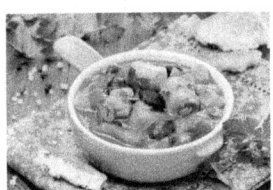

Preparation Time: 10 Minutes
Cooking Time: 30 Minutes
Servings: 4
Ingredients
- 1-pound white fish fillets, boneless, skinless, and cubed
- 2 tomatoes, cubed
- 1 avocado, pitted and chopped
- 1 tablespoon oregano, chopped
- 1 tablespoon parsley, chopped
- 1 red onion, sliced
- 1 teaspoon sweet paprika
- 2 tablespoons olive oil
- A pinch of salt and black pepper
- Juice of 1 lime
- 1 cup chicken stock

Preparation

1. Warm-up oil in a pot over medium heat, add the onion and sauté within 5 minutes.

2. Add the fish, the avocado, and the other ingredients, toss, cook over medium heat for 25 minutes more.

3. Once done, divide into bowls and serve for dinner.

Nutritional Info

Calories: 78, Carbohydrates: 8g, Fat: 1g, Protein: 11g, Sodium: 151 mg

49

TURKEY BREAST WITH COCONUT AND ZUCCHINI

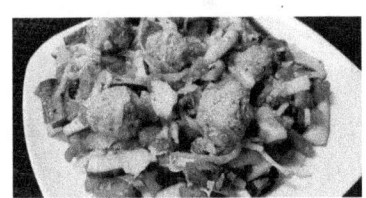

Preparation Time: 10 Minutes
Cooking Time: 30 Minutes
Servings: 4
Ingredients:
- 2 garlic cloves, minced
- 1-pound turkey breast, skinless, boneless, and cubed
- black pepper
- 1 yellow onion, chopped
- 2 tablespoons olive oil
- 1 zucchini, sliced
- A pinch of sea salt
- 1 cup coconut cream

Preparation
1. Bring the pan to medium heat, add the onion and the garlic and sauté for 5 minutes.
2. Put the meat and brown within 5 minutes more.
3. Add the rest of the ingredients, toss, bring to a simmer and cook over medium heat for 20 minutes more.
4. Serve for lunch.

Nutritional Info

Calories 200, Fat 4g, Fibre 2g, Sodium 111mg, Carbohydrates 14g, Protein 7g

50

CREAMY PUMPKIN PASTA

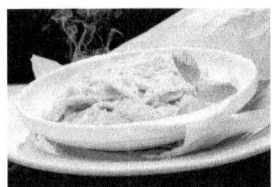

Preparation Time: 15 Minutes
Cooking Time: 30 Minutes
Servings: 6
Ingredients:
- 1-pound whole-grain linguine
- ¼ teaspoon ground cayenne pepper
- garlic cloves, peeled and minced
- 2 tablespoons chopped fresh sage 1½ cups pumpkin purée
- ¾ teaspoon kosher or sea salt
- cup unsalted vegetable stock
- ½ cup freshly grated Parmesan cheese, divided
- ½ teaspoon ground nutmeg
- ½ teaspoon ground black pepper
- 1 tablespoon olive oil
- ½ cup low-fat evaporated milk

Preparation

1. Cook the whole-grain linguine in a large pot of boiled water. Reserve ½ cup of pasta water and drain the rest. Set the pasta aside.

2. Heat-up olive oil over medium heat in a large skillet. Add

the garlic and sage and sauté for 1 to 2 minutes, until soft and fragrant.

3. Whisk in the pumpkin purée, stock, milk, and reserved pasta water and simmer for 4 to 5 minutes, until thickened.

4. Whisk in the salt, black pepper, nutmeg, and cayenne pepper and half of the Parmesan cheese. Stir in the cooked wholegrain linguine.

5. Evenly divide the pasta into 6 bowls and top with the remaining Parmesan cheese.

Nutritional Info

Calories: 381, Fat: 8g, Carbohydrate: 63g, Protein: 15g, Sodium: 175mg

51
TASTY ROASTED BROCCOLI

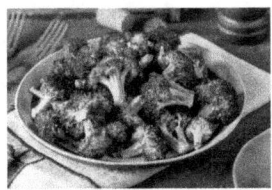

Preparation Time: 5 Minutes
Cooking Time: 20 Minutes
Serving: 4
Ingredients:
- Sunflower seeds and pepper to taste
- 1 tablespoon olive oil
- 4 cups broccoli florets

Preparation
1. Pre-heat your oven to 400 degrees F.
2. Add broccoli in a zip bag alongside oil and shake until coated.
3. Add seasoning and shake again.
4. Spread broccoli out on a baking sheet, bake for 20 minutes.
5. Let it cool and serve. Enjoy!

Nutritional Info
Calories: 62, Fat: 4g, Carbohydrates: 4g, Protein: 4g

52

LIME SHRIMP AND KALE

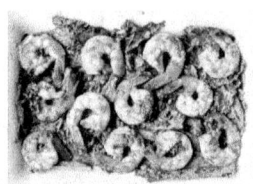

Preparation Time: 10 Minutes
Cooking Time: 20 Minutes
Servings: 4
Ingredients:
- 1-pound shrimp, peeled and deveined
- 1 teaspoon sweet paprika
- 1 tablespoon olive oil
- 2 tablespoons parsley, chopped
- Zest of 1 lime, grated
- 4 scallions, chopped
- A pinch of salt and black pepper
- Juice of 1 lime

Preparation

1. Bring the pan to medium heat, add the scallions and sauté for 5 minutes.
2. Add the shrimp and the other ingredients, toss, cook over medium heat for 15 minutes more, divide into bowls and serve.

Nutritional Info

Calories: 149, Carbohydrates: 12g, Sodium: 250 mg, Fat: 4g, Protein: 21g

53

CHICKEN SALSA

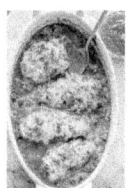

Preparation Time: 4 minutes

Cooking Time: 14 minutes

Serving: 1

Ingredients:
- 2 chicken breasts
- 1 cup plain Greek Yogurt
- ½ cup of kite cashew cheese, cubed
- 1 taco seasoning mix
- 1 cup salsa

Preparation

1. Take a skillet and place over average heat.
2. Add in chicken breast, ½ cup of salsa, and taco seasoning.
3. Mix well and cook for 12-15 minutes until the chicken is done.
4. Take the chicken out and cube them.
5. Place the cubes on a toothpick and top with cheddar.
6. Place yogurt and remaining salsa in cups and use as dips. Enjoy!

Nutritional Info

Calories: 359 Protein: 43g Carbohydrates: 14g Fat: 14g

54

VEGETARIAN LASAGNA

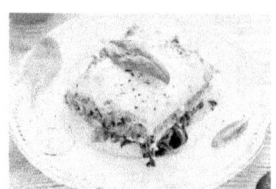

Preparation Time: 15 Minutes
Cooking Time: 30 Minutes
Servings: 6
Ingredients:
- 1 cup low-sodium vegetable broth
- ½ cup bell pepper, diced
- 1 cup carrot, diced
- 1 eggplant, sliced
- 1 cup spinach, chopped
- 1 cup tomatoes, chopped
- 4 oz low-fat cottage cheese
- 1 teaspoon chili powder
- 1 tablespoon olive oil

Preparation

1. Put carrot, bell pepper, and spinach in the saucepan. Add olive oil and chili powder and stir the vegetables well. Cook them for 5 minutes.

2. Make the sliced eggplant layer in the casserole mold and top it with vegetable mixture.

3. Add tomatoes, vegetable stock, and cottage cheese. Bake the lasagna for 30 minutes at 375F.

Nutritional Info

Calories 77, Protein 4.1g, Sodium 124mg, Fat 3g, Carbohydrates 9.7g

55

CARROT CAKES

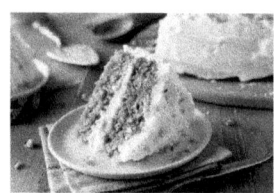

Preparation Time: 15 Minutes
Cooking Time: 10 Minutes
Servings: 4
Ingredients:
- 1 cup carrot, grated
- 1 egg, beaten
- 1 tablespoon semolina
- 1 teaspoon Italian seasonings
- 1 tablespoon sesame oil

Preparation

1. In the mixing bowl, mix up grated carrot, semolina, egg, and Italian seasonings.

2. Heat sesame oil in the skillet. Make the carrot cakes with the help of 2 spoons and put them in the skillet. Roast the cakes for 4 minutes per side.

Nutritional Info

Calories 70, Carbohydrates 4.8g, Protein 1.9g, Fat 4.9g, Sodium 35mg

56
CHIPOTLE LETTUCE CHICKEN

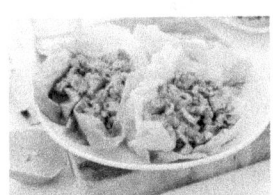

Preparation Time: 10 minutes
Cooking Time: 25 minutes
Serving: 6
Ingredients
- 1 pound chicken breast, cut into strips
- Fresh tomato slices for garnish
- 1 red onion, finely sliced
- Lettuce as needed
- 1 teaspoon chipotle, chopped
- Lime wedges
- Fresh coriander leaves
- 14 ounces tomatoes
- Splash of olive oil
- Jalapeno chilies, sliced
- ½ teaspoon cumin

Preparation
1. Take a non-stick frying pan and place it over medium heat.
2. Add oil and heat it up.
3. Add chicken and cook until brown.
4. Keep the chicken on the side.

5. Add tomatoes, sugar, chipotle, cumin to the same pan and simmer for 25 minutes until you have a nice sauce.

6. Add chicken into the sauce and cook for 5 minutes.

7. Transfer the mix to another place.

8. Use lettuce wraps to take a portion of the mixture and serve with a squeeze of lemon. Enjoy!

Nutritional Info

Calories: 332, Protein: 34g, Fat: 15g, Carbohydrates: 13g

57
VEGAN CHILI

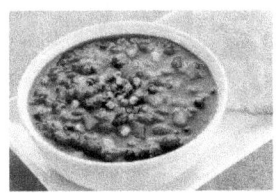

Preparation Time: 15 Minutes
Cooking Time: 25 Minutes
Servings: 4
Ingredients:
- (1) 15-oz can red kidney beans, cooked
- ½ cup bulgur
- 1 cup tomatoes, chopped
- 1 chili pepper, chopped
- 1 teaspoon tomato paste
- ½ cup celery stalk, chopped
- 1 cup low-sodium vegetable broth

Preparation

Put all ingredients in the big saucepan and stir well. Close the lid and simmer the chili for 25 minutes over medium-low heat.

Nutritional Info

Calories 234 Protein 13.1g Carbohydrates 44.9g Fat 0.9g Sodium 92mg

58

FRUITED QUINOA SALAD

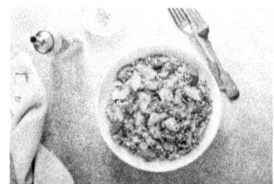

Preparation Time: 15 Minutes
Cooking Time: 15 Minutes
Servings: 2
Ingredients
- 2 cups cooked quinoa
- ½ cup blueberries
- 1 cup strawberry, quartered
- 1 tablespoon pine nuts Chopped
- mint leaves for garnish Lemon vinaigrette:
- 1 mango, sliced and peeled
- ¼ cup olive oil
- Zest 1 lemon
- 3 tablespoons lemon juice
- 1 teaspoon sugar
- ¼ cup apple cider vinegar

Preparation

1. For the Lemon Vinaigrette, whisk olive oil, apple cider vinegar, lemon zest and juice, and sugar to a container; set aside.

2. Combine quinoa, mango strawberries, blueberries, and pine nuts in a large container.

3.Stir the lemon vinaigrette and garnish with mint.

4.Serve and enjoy!

Nutritional Info

Calories 425, Sodium 16mg, Carbohydrates 76.1g, Proteins 11.3g, Fat 10.9

59
CHUNKY TOMATOES

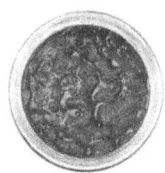

Preparation Time: 15 Minutes

Cooking Time: 15 Minutes

Servings: 3

Ingredients

- 6 cups plum tomatoes, roughly chopped
- 1 teaspoon Italian seasonings
- ½ cup onion, diced
- 1 teaspoon canola oil
- ½ teaspoon garlic, diced
- ¼ teaspoon chili pepper, chopped

Preparation

1. Heat canola oil in the saucepan. Add chili pepper and onion. Cook the vegetables for 5 minutes.

2. Stir them from time to time. After this, add tomatoes, garlic, and Italian seasonings. Close the lid and sauté the dish for 10 minutes.

Nutritional Info

Calories 550, Protein 1.7g, Sodium 17mg, Carbohydrates 8.4g, Fat 2.3g

60

CAULIFLOWER BREAD STICK

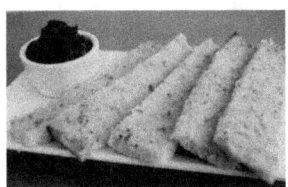

Preparation Time: 10 Minutes
Cooking Time: 48 Minutes
Serving: 5
Ingredients:
- 1 cup cashew cheese/ kite ricotta cheese
- ½ teaspoon Italian seasoning
- ¼ teaspoon red pepper flakes
- Parmesan cheese, grated
- 1/8 teaspoon kosher sunflower seeds
- 1 tablespoon organic almond butter
- 2 cups cauliflower rice, cooked for 3 minutes in a microwave
- 3 teaspoons garlic, minced
- 1 whole egg

Preparation
1. Pre-heat your oven to 350 degrees F.
2. Add almond butter in a small pan and melt over low heat
3. Add red pepper flakes, garlic to the almond butter and cook for 2-3 minutes.
4. Add garlic and almond butter mix to the bowl with cooked cauliflower and add the Italian seasoning.

5. Season with sunflower seeds and mix, refrigerate for 10 minutes.

6. Add cheese and eggs to the bowl and mix.

7. Place a layer of parchment paper at the bottom of a 9 x 9 baking dish and grease with cooking spray, add egg and mozzarella cheese mix to the cauliflower mix.

8. Add mix to the pan and smooth to a thin layer with the palms of your hand.

9. Bake for 30 minutes, take out from the oven, and top with few shakes of parmesan and mozzarella.

10. Cook for 8 minutes more. Enjoy!

Nutritional Info

Carbohydrates: 11.5g, Fibre: 2g, Protein: 10.7g, Fat: 20g

SNACKS

61
AVOCADO GUACAMOLE

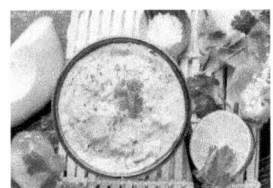

Preparation time: 10 minutes

Servings: 4

Ingredients
- 2 medium ripe avocados
- 1 Serrano pepper
- 1 tomato
- 1 small red onion
- 2 tbsp. fresh cilantro leaves
- 1 tbsp. fresh lime juice
- 1 garlic clove
- Pinch of salt

Preparation

1. In a large container, add avocado and mash it completely with a fork.

2. Add what of left of the ingredients and gently stir to combine.

3. Serve immediately.

Nutritional Info

Calories: 217, Fat: 19.7g, Carbohydrates: 11.3g, Fibre: 7.4g, Sugar: 1.7g, Protein: 2.3g, Sodium: 47mg

62

SAVOURY STUFFED MUSHROOMS

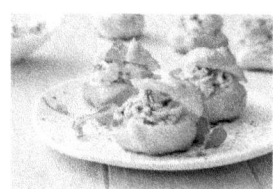

Preparation Time: 10 Minutes
Cooking Time: 15 Minutes
Servings: 6

Ingredients
- 16 ounces' fresh mushrooms
- 2 Tbsp. Olive oil
- ½ cup Salt-free bread crumbs
- 1 tsp. dried Italian seasoning
- 1 Egg white
- ½ tsp. ground black pepper
- 4 cloves Garlic
- ½ cup Shredded Swiss cheese

Preparation
1. Preheat the oven to 400F. Spray a baking sheet with oil.
2. Remove stems from the mushrooms and keep caps intact.
3. Place mushroom stems in a food processor and add the remaining ingredients. Pulse to combine.
4. Stuff each mushroom cap with the mixture.
5. Place the mushrooms in the baking sheet and place the sheet in the oven.

6.Bake for 15 minutes. Serve.

Nutritional Info

Calories: 124, Fat: 7g, Carbohydrates: 10g, Protein: 5g, Sodium 30mg

63

PEAS & FETA SANDWICH

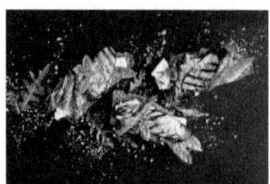

Preparation Time: 10 Minutes
Servings: 4
Ingredients
- 1 cup boiled peas
- 1 tbsp. fresh lemon juice
- ½ cups feta cheese
- 8 whole-wheat bread slices
- 2 tbsp. fresh mint leaves
- 1 tbsp. olive oil

Preparation

1. In a bowl, mix together peas, oil, feta, lemon juice, mint, Pinch of salt pepper.

2. Spread the peas mixture over 4 bread slices evenly. Cover with remaining 4 bread slices. With a knife, carefully cut the sandwiches diagonally and serve.

Nutritional Info

Calories: 235, Fat: 9.4g, Carbohydrates: 27g, Fibre: 5.5g, Sugar: 5.7g, Protein: 11.2g, Sodium: 350mg

64

CRUSTED CHICKEN WITH DIPPING SAUCE

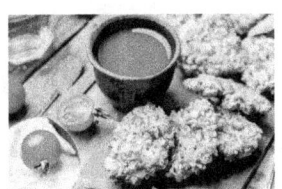

Preparation Time: 10 Minutes
Cooking Time: 20 Minutes
Servings: 6

Ingredients
- 2 Tbsp. orange marmalade
- 4 Boneless, skinless chicken thighs
- ¼ cup unsweetened coconut
- 1 Egg white
- 1 tsp. garlic powder
- Cooking spray to grease the baking sheet
- ¼ tsp. ground black pepper
- ¼ cup Salt-free bread crumbs
- 1 ½ tsp. unflavoured rice vinegar
- ¼ tsp. Dried red pepper flakes

Preparation
1. Preheat the oven to 425F.
2. Cut chicken into bite-sized pieces.
3. In a bowl, add coconut, bread crumbs, garlic powder, and black pepper and mix well.
4. Beat the egg white in a bowl.

5. Submerge each piece of chicken into the egg, then coat with bread crumbs.

6. Place on a prepared baking sheet.

7. Bake for 10 minutes.

8. Flip chicken and cook another 10 minutes more.

9. Meanwhile, in a bowl, add the vinegar, marmalade, and red pepper flakes, and stir well.

10. Serve the chicken with dipping sauce.

Nutritional Info

Calories: 105, Fat: 4g, Carbohydrates: 10g, Protein: 7g, Sodium 39mg

65
YOGURT & BANANA BOWL

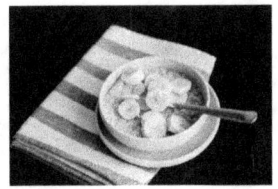

Preparation Time: 10 Minutes
Servings: 2
Ingredients
- 1 banana, peeled and mashed
- 2 tbsp. wheat germ, divided
- 1 cup fat-free plain Greek yogurt

Preparation
In a bowl, add yogurt, banana, and wheat germ and stir to combine. Serve immediately.

Nutritional Info
Calories: 135, Fat: 1.1g, Carbohydrates: 25.4g, Fibre: 2.6g, Sugar: 7.8g, Protein: 7.7g, Sodium: 87mg

66

ZUCCHINI STICKS

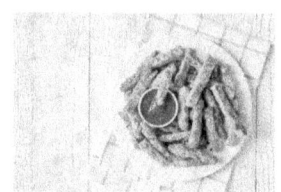

Preparation Time: 10 Minutes

Cooking Time: 15 Minutes

Servings: 6

Ingredients

- 2 Medium zucchinis, cut into 16 equal wedges
- ¼ tsp. freshly ground black pepper
- 1 Tbsp. Water
- 1 Tbsp. grated Parmesan cheese
- 1 Egg white
- 1 tsp. dried Italian seasoning
- ½ cup No-salt-added pasta sauce
- 3 Tbsp. salt-free bread crumbs
- ½ tsp. onion powder
- 1/8 tsp. ground sweet paprika
- ½ tsp. garlic powder

Preparation

1. Preheat the oven to 450F. Spray a baking sheet with oil.
2. Beat the egg whites and water in a bowl.
3. In another bowl, place bread crumbs, cheese, and seasonings and whisk to combine.

4. Dip each piece of zucchini into the egg.
5. Then roll in bread crumbs.
6. Place on the baking sheet and bake for 15 minutes.
7. Meanwhile, warm the pasta sauce on the stovetop.
8. Serve zucchini stick with warm sauce.

Nutritional Info

Calories: 39, Fat: 1g, Carbohydrates: 6g, Protein: 2g, Sodium 28mg

67

YOGURT & DRIED FRUIT BARS

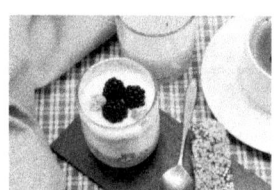

Preparation Time: 10 Minutes
Cooking Time: 25 Minutes
Servings: 8
Ingredients
- 1 cup fat-free plain yogurt
- 1 (6-oz.) package mixed dried fruit
- 1 large egg
- 1½ cups whole-wheat flour
- ½ tsp. ground ginger
- 1/3 cups unsalted walnuts
- 1 tsp. ground cinnamon
- 1 tsp. baking soda
- ½ tsp. organic baking powder

Preparation

1. Preheat the oven to 350 °F. Lightly grease an 8-inch baking dish.

2. In a large container, add all ingredients and mix until well combined. Transfer the mix into the prepared baking dish evenly and with the back of a spatula, smooth the top surface.

3. Bake for about 25 minutes.

4. Take out of the oven and set aside to cool completely.
5. With a sharp knife, cut into 8 equal-sized bars and serve.

Nutritional Info

Calories: 245, Fat: 7.7g, Carbohydrates: 40.1g, Fibre: 2.2g, Sugar: 17.4g, Protein: 5.3g, Sodium: 150mg

68

SALT-FREE PICKLES

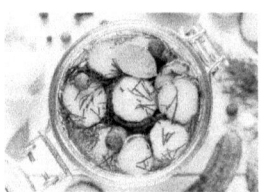

Preparation Time: 10 Minutes

Cooking Time: 5 Minutes

Servings: 40

Ingredients

- 1 tsp. Dried red pepper flakes
- 3 Large cucumbers
- 2 cups Sugar
- ½ tsp. Whole peppercorns
- 1 Onion
- 3 Bay leaves
- 4 cups While vinegar
- 1 Tbsp. Mustard seed
- 6 cloves Garlic

Preparation

1. Slice the cucumbers into thin rounds.
2. Place the cucumber, onion, and minced garlic in a jar.
3. Add the remaining ingredients in a saucepan. Stir and bring to a boil.
4. Once boiling, pour over the mixture in a jar.

5. Cover with the lid and let sit until cool.
6. Serve.

Nutritional Info

Calories: 23, Fat: 0g, Carbohydrates: 4g, Protein: 0g, Sodium 2mg

69

OATMEAL COOKIES

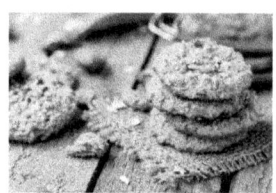

Preparation Time: 15 Minutes
Cooking Time: 12 Minutes
Servings: 18
Ingredients
- 2 cups quick oats
- 2 tsp. chia seeds
- 1 large apple
- ½ tsp. ground cinnamon
- ¼ cups raisins
- 1 tsp. apple cider vinegar
- 4 Medjool dates
- ½ tsp. baking soda
- ¼ tsp. ground nutmeg
- ¼ tsp. ground ginger
- 2 tbsp. cold water
- ¼ cups warm filtered water

Preparation

1. Preheat the oven to 375F. Line a large cookie sheet with a large greased parchment paper.

2.In a bowl, mix together warm water and chia seeds. Set aside until thickened.

3.In a large food processor, add 1 cup of the oats and pulse until finely ground. Transfer the ground oats in a large bowl. Add the remaining oats, baking soda, spices, and raisins and mix well.

4.Now in the blender, add the remaining ingredients and pulse until smooth. Transfer the apple mixture into the bowl with oat mixture and mix well.

5.Add the chia seeds mixture and stir to combine. Spoon the mixture onto the prepared cookie sheet in a single layer and with your finger, flatten each cookie slightly.

6.Bake until golden brown or for about 12 minutes. Remove from the oven and place the cookie sheet onto a wire rack to cool for about 5 minutes.

7.Invert the cookies onto the wire rack to cool before serving.

Nutritional Info

Calories: 68, Fat: 0.8g, Carbohydrates: 14.5g, Fibre: 2g, Sugar: 6.6g, Protein: 1.6g, Sodium: 37 mg

70
CHEESY POPCORN

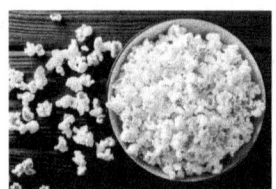

Preparation time: 5 minutes
Cooking time: 2 minutes
Servings: 10
Ingredients
- 2 Tbsp. Nutritional yeast flakes
- ½ cup Popcorn kernels
- 2 tsp. Olive oil
- ¾ tsp. Onion powder
- 1 tsp. Dried parsley
- 1 ½ tsp. Dried dill
- ¼ tsp. Ground black pepper
- ½ tsp. Ground sweet paprika
- ¾ tsp. Garlic powder
- ¼ tsp. Dried thyme

Preparation

1. In a bowl, add yeast, dill, parsley, garlic powder, onion powder, paprika, thyme, and black pepper. Mix well.
2. Place popcorn kernels into an air popper.
3. Place a stockpot beneath the popcorn dispenser.

4. Turn the appliance on, and wait until kernels have popped. Turn off the popper and set it aside.

5. Drizzle the oil over popcorn and toss to coat. Then sprinkle with seasoning mixture and mix to coat. Serve.

Nutritional Info

Calories: 55, Fat: 1g, Carbohydrates: 8g, Protein: 2g, Sodium 2mg

71

ROASTED HARISSA CARROTS

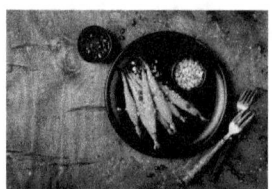

Preparation Time: 10 Minutes
Cooking Time: 15 Minutes
Serves 4
Ingredients
- 2 tablespoons harissa
- 1-pound carrots, peeled and sliced into 1-inch-thick rounds
- 2 tablespoons extra-virgin olive oil
- 1 teaspoon ground cumin
- 1 teaspoon honey
- ½ cup fresh parsley, chopped
- ½ teaspoon kosher salt

Preparation

1. Preheat the oven to 450°F. Line a baking sheet with parchment paper or foil.
2. In a large container, combine the carrots, olive oil, harissa, honey, cumin, and salt.
3. Arrange in a solo layer on the baking sheet. Roast for 15 minutes.
4. Remove from the oven, add the parsley, and toss together.

Nutritional Info
Calories: 120; fat: 8g; Sodium: 255mg; Carbohydrates: 13g; Fibre: 4g; Sugars: 7g; Protein: 1g

72

CHOCOLATE COCONUT BOMBS

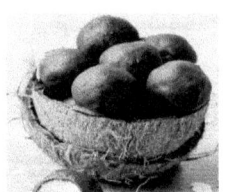

Preparation Time: 20 Minutes
Cooking Time: 20 Minutes
Servings: 12
Ingredients:
- ½ cup dark cocoa powder
- 1 cup coconut oil, solid
- 5 drops stevia
- 1 tablespoon peppermint extract
- ½ tablespoon vanilla extract

Preparation

1. In a high-speed food processor and add all the ingredients. Blend until combined.

2. Take a teaspoon and drop a spoonful onto parchment paper. Refrigerate until solidified and keep refrigerated.

Nutritional Info

Calories: 126 Carbohydrates: 0g Fibre: 0g Protein: 0g Fat: 14g Sodium: 30 mg

73
KALE CHIPS

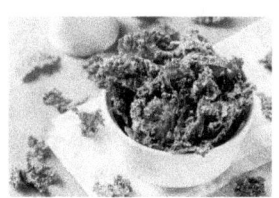

Preparation Time: 10 Minutes
Cooking Time: 12 Minutes
Servings: 6
Ingredients
- 1 large bunch Kale
- ¼ tsp. Sea salt
- 1 Tbsp. Olive oil

Preparation

1. Preheat the oven to 350F. Line a cookie sheet with parchment paper.
2. Spread kale out on the baking sheet and drizzle with olive oil and season with salt.
3. Bake for 10 to 12 minutes.

Nutritional info
Calories: 110, Sodium 210mg, Fat: 5g, Carb: 16g, Protein: 5g

74

APPLE DUMPLINGS

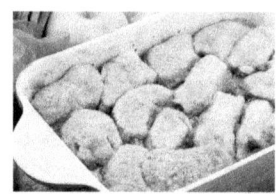

Preparation Time: 10 Minutes
Cooking Time: 30 Minutes
Servings: 6
Ingredients:
Dough:
- 1 tablespoon butter
- 2 tablespoons brandy or apple liquor
- 1 teaspoon honey
- 2 tablespoons rolled oats
- 2 tablespoons buckwheat flour
- 1 cup whole-wheat flour

Apple filling:
- 6 large tart apples, thinly sliced
- Zest of one lemon
- 2 tablespoons honey
- 1 teaspoon nutmeg

Preparation
1. Warm oven to heat at 350 degrees F.
2. Combine flours with oats, honey, and butter in a food processor. Pulse this mixture for few times, then stirs in apple

liquor or brandy. Mix until it forms a ball. Wrap it in a plastic sheet.

3. Refrigerate for 2 hours. Mix apples with honey, nutmeg, and lemon zest, then set it aside. Spread the dough into ¼ inch thick sheet.

4. Cut it into 8-inch circles and layer the greased muffin cups with the dough circles.

5. Divide the apple mixture into the muffin cups and seal the dough from the top. Bake for 30 minutes at 350 degrees F until golden brown. Enjoy.

Nutritional Info

Calories 178 Fat 5.7 g Sodium 114 mg carbohydrate 12.4 g Protein 9.1 g

75

ROASTED CHICKPEAS

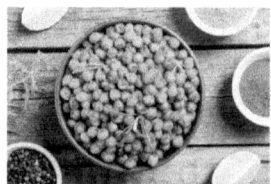

Preparation Time: 10 Minutes
Cooking Time: 45 Minutes
Servings: 12
Ingredients
- 4 C. cooked chickpeas
- 2 garlic cloves, minced
- ¼ tsp. ground cumin
- 1 tbsp. olive oil
- ½ tsp. dried oregano, crushed
- ½ tsp. smoked paprika

Preparation

1. Preheat the oven to 400 °F. Grease a large baking sheet.
2. Place chickpeas onto the prepared baking sheet in a single layer. Roast for about 30 minutes, stir the chickpeas after every 10 minutes.
3. Meanwhile, in a small mixing container, mix together garlic, thyme, and spices. Remove the baking sheet from the oven.
4. Place the garlic mixture and oil over the chickpeas and toss to coat well. Roast for about 10-15 minutes more.

5. Now, turn the oven off but leave the baking sheet inside for about 10 minutes before serving.

Nutritional Info

Calories: 92, Sodium: 10mg, Fat: 1.9g, Carbohydrates: 15g, Fibre: 0.1g, Protein: 4.1g

DESSERTS

76

FROZEN MANGO TREAT

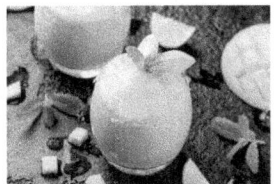

Preparation time: 10 minutes
Servings: 4
Ingredients
- 1 tbsp. fresh mint leaves
- ½ C. chilled water
- 2 tbsp. fresh lime juice
- 1 tbsp. fresh mint leaves
- 3 C. frozen mango, peeled, pitted, and chopped

Preparation

1. In a high-velocity blender, add all ingredients and pulse until smooth.
2. Transfer into serving bowls and serve immediately.

Nutritional info:
Calories: 76, Fat: 0.5g, Carbohydrates: 18.7g, Fibre: 2.1g, Sugar: 16.9g, Protein: 1.1g, Sodium: 3mg

77

PUMPKIN WITH CHIA SEEDS PUDDING

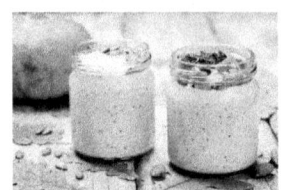

Preparation Time: 60 Minutes

Cooking Time: 0 Minutes

Servings: 4

Ingredients:

For the Pudding:
- ½ cup organic chia seeds
- 1 ¼ cup low-fat milk
- ¼ cup raw maple syrup
- 1 cup pumpkin puree extract

For the Toppings:
- ¼ cup organic sunflower seeds
- ¼ cup blueberries
- ¼ cup coarsely chopped almonds

Preparation

1. Add all the ingredients for the pudding in a bowl and mix until blended.

2. Cover and store in a chiller for 1-hour.

3. Remove from the chiller, transfer contents to a jar and add the ingredients for the toppings.

4. Serve immediately.

Nutritional Info

Calories 189 Sodium 42 mg Fats 7 g Carbohydrates 27 g Fibres 4 g Proteins 5 g Sugar 18 g

78

GRILLED PINEAPPLE STRIPS

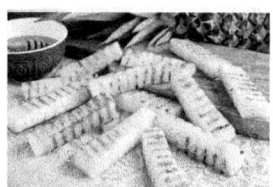

Preparation Time: 15 Minutes
Cooking Time: 5 Minutes
Servings: 6
Ingredients:
- 1 pineapple
- 3 tablespoons brown sugar
- 1 tablespoon raw honey
- 1 dash of iodized salt
- Vegetable oil
- 1 tablespoon olive oil
- 1 tablespoon lime juice extract

Preparation

1. Peel the pineapple, remove the eyes of the fruit, and discard the core.
2. Slice the pineapple lengthwise, forming six wedges.
3. Brush the coating mixture on the pineapple. Grease an oven or outdoor grill rack with vegetable oil.
4. Place the pineapple wedges on the grill rack and heat for a few minutes per side until golden brownish, basting it frequently with a reserved glaze. Serve on a platter.

Nutrition info:

Calories 97 Fats 2 g Carbohydrates 20 g Proteins 1 g Fibres 1 g Sugar 17 g Sodium 2 mg

79

PEACH SORBET

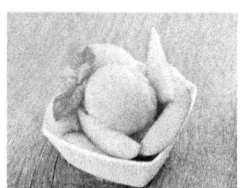

Preparation Time: 10 Minutes

Servings: 6

Ingredients:

- 6 medium peaches, pitted and chopped
- 3 tbsp. unsalted almonds, chopped
- 1¾ C. unsweetened coconut milk
- ¼ tsp. ground cinnamon
- 1 tsp. organic vanilla extract

Preparation

1. In a blender, add peaches and pulse until a puree form.

2. Add what is left, the ingredients, and pulse until smooth and creamy.

3. Transfer the peach mixture into an ice-cream maker and process according to the manufacturer's directions.

4. Now, transfer into an airtight container and freeze for 4-5 hours or until set completely. Top with an apple slice and serve.

Nutritional info:

Calories: 92, Fat: 3.1g, Carbohydrates: 15g, Fibre: 3g, Sugar: 14.2g, Protein: 2g, Sodium: 20mg

80

CHOCO BANANA CAKE

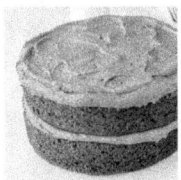

Preparation Time: 15 Minutes
Cooking Time: 30 Minutes
Servings: 18
Ingredients:
- ½ cup semisweet dark chocolate
- ½ cup brown sugar
- ½ teaspoon baking soda
- 1 tablespoon lemon juice extract
- 1 cup all-purpose flour
- ¼ cup unsweetened cocoa powder
- ¼ cup canola oil
- 1 large egg
- 1 egg white
- ¾ cup soymilk
- 1 large, ripe, mashed banana
- 1 teaspoon vanilla extract

Preparation

1. Preheat the oven to 350 °F. Coat a baking pan with a non-stick spray. Whisk brown sugar, flour, baking soda, and cocoa powder in a container.

2. In another container, whisk bananas, lemon juice extract, vanilla extract, oil, soymilk, egg, and egg whites.

3. Create a hole in the flour mixture's core or centre, then pour in the banana mixture and mix in the dark chocolate.

4. Stir all the fixing with a spoon until thoroughly blended; spoon the batter onto the baking pan.

5. Place in the oven and bake within 25-30 minutes until the centre springs back when pressed lightly using your fingertips.

Nutritional info:

Calories 150 Sodium 52 mg Cholesterol 12 mg Carbohydrates 27 g Proteins 3 g Fats 3 g

81

HERBED GROUND CHICKEN

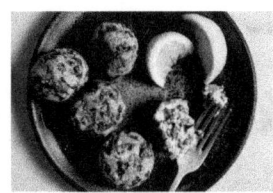

Preparation Time: 10 Minutes
Cooking Time: 15 Minutes
Servings: 4
Ingredients:
- 1 lb. lean ground chicken
- 4 garlic cloves, minced
- 1 tsp. unsweetened applesauce
- ½ tsp. fresh ginger, minced
- 1 Pinch of salt
- 1 tbsp. fresh lime juice
- 2 tbsp. olive oil
- 2 shallots, chopped finely
- Freshly ground black pepper, to taste
- 2 jalapeño peppers, seeded
- ½ C. fresh basil, chopped

Preparation:

1. In a large skillet with oil over medium heat, apply heat and sauté shallots for about 2-3 minutes.

2. Add garlic and ginger and sauté for about 1 minute. Add chicken and cook for about 5-7minutes.

3. Stir in applesauce and cook for about 3-4 minutes, stirring occasionally.

4. Stir in remaining ingredients and remove from heat. Serve hot.

Nutritional info:

Calories: 227, Fat: 13.2g, Carbohydrates: 3.6g, Fibre: 0.5g, Sugar: 0.4g, Protein: 23.7g, Sodium: 225mg

82

ZESTY ZUCCHINI MUFFINS

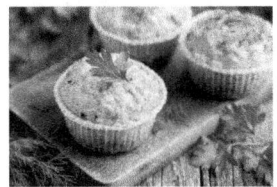

Preparation Time: 15 Minutes
Cooking Time: 30 Minutes
Servings: 12
Ingredients:
- Vegetable oil cooking spray
- ½ cup of sugar
- ¼ teaspoon iodized salt
- ¼ teaspoon ground nutmeg
- ¾ cup skim milk
- 1 cup shredded zucchini
- 1 tablespoon baking powder
- 1 large egg
- 2 teaspoons grated lemon rind
- 2 cups of all-purpose flour
- 3 tablespoons vegetable oil

Preparation:

1. Mix the flour, baking powder, sugar, salt, plus lemon rinds in a bowl. Create a well in the centre of the flour batter.

2. In another container, mix zucchini, milk, vegetable oil, and egg. Coat muffin cups with vegetable oil cooking spray.

3. Divide the batter equally into 12 muffin cups. Transfer the muffin cups to the baking pan, put it in a microwave oven, and bake at 400 °F within 30 minutes until light golden brown.

4. Remove, then allow to cool on a wire rack before serving.

Nutritional info:

Proteins 0 g, Calories 169, Sodium 211.5 mg, Carbohydrates 29.1 g, Fats 4.8 g, Fibres 2.5 g

83

MANGO RICE PUDDING

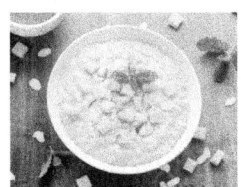

Preparation Time: 15 Minutes

Cooking Time: 35 Minutes

Servings: 4

Ingredients:

- ½ teaspoon ground cinnamon
- ¼ teaspoon iodized salt
- 1 teaspoon vanilla extract
- 1 cup long-grain uncooked brown rice
- 2 mediums ripe, peeled, cored mango
- 1 cup vanilla soymilk
- 1 tablespoon sugar
- 2 cups of water

Preparation:

1. Bring saltwater to a boil in a saucepan to cook rice; after a few minutes, simmer covered within 30-35 minutes until the rice absorbs the water.

2. Mash the mango with a mortar and pestle or stainless-steel fork.

3. Pour milk, sugar, cinnamon, and the mashed mango into the rice; cook uncovered on low heat, stirring frequently.

4. Remove the mango rice pudding from the heat, then stir in the vanilla soymilk. Serve immediately.

Nutritional info:

Calories 275 Sodium 176 mg Carbohydrates 58 mg Sugar 20 g Fats 3 g Fibres 3 g

84

CHICKEN MEATLOAF

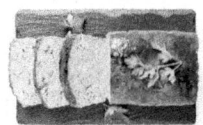

Preparation Time: 15 Minutes
Cooking Time: 1¼ Hours
Servings: 4
Ingredients:
- ½ C. cooked chickpeas, rinsed and drained
- Freshly ground black pepper, to taste
- 1 C. red bell pepper, seeded and minced
- 1/3 C. steel-cut oats
- 2 tbsp. dried onion flakes, crushed
- 2 egg whites
- 10 oz. lean ground chicken
- 1 C. celery stalk, minced
- 1 C. tomato puree, divided
- 1 tbsp. prepared mustard

Preparation;
1. Preheat the oven to 350 °F. Grease a 9x5-inch loaf pan.
2. In a food processor, add chickpeas, egg whites, and black pepper and pulse until smooth.
3. Transfer the chickpea mixture into a large container. Add

chicken, bell pepper, celery, oats, ½ C. of tomato puree, and onion flakes and mix until well combined.

4. Transfer the mixture into the prepared loaf pan evenly and with the back of a spoon, smooth the surface.

5. In a container, mix together mustard and remaining tomato puree. Spread tomato puree mixture over loaf evenly.

6. Bake for about 1¼ hours. Pull from oven and set aside for 5-10 minutes before serving.

7. Carefully remove from loaf pan. With a sharp knife, cut the loaf into desired sized slices and serve.

Nutritional info:

Calories: 300, Fat: 7.2g, Carbohydrates: 30g, Fibre: 8.3g, Sugar: 8g, Protein: 25.4g, Sodium: 180mg

85

BLUEBERRY OAT MUFFINS

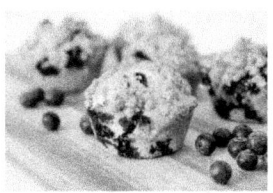

Preparation Time: 15 Minutes

Cooking Time: 30 Minutes

Servings: 12

Ingredients:

- ½ cup raw oatmeal
- ½ teaspoon baking powder
- ½ teaspoon iodized salt
- ½ cup dry milk
- ¼ cup of vegetable oil
- ¼ teaspoon baking soda
- 1/3 cup sugar
- 1 ½ cup flour
- 1 cup milk
- 1 cup blueberries

Preparation:

1. Preheat oven to 350 °F. Coat the muffin tins with vegetable oil.

2. Mix or combine the flour, baking soda, baking powder, oats, sugar, and salt in a bowl. Mix milk, dry milk, egg, and vegetable oil in another container.

3. Pour the container of wet fixing into the bowl of dry fixing and mix partially.

4. Add the blueberries and mix until the consistency turns lumpy. Scoop blueberry batter into the muffin tins.

5. Bake within 30 minutes until the muffins turn golden brown on the edges.

6. Serve warm immediately or put it in an airtight container and store it in the refrigerator to chill.

Nutritional info:

Calories 150 Sodium 180 mg Carbohydrates 22 g Proteins 4 g Fats 5 g Fibres 1 g

86

RASPBERRY PEACH PANCAKE

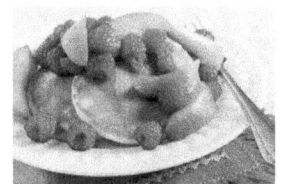

Preparation Time: 15 Minutes
Cooking Time: 30 Minutes
Servings: 4
Ingredients:
- ½ teaspoon sugar
- ½ cup raspberries
- ½ cup fat-free milk
- ½ cup all-purpose flour
- ¼ cup vanilla yogurt
- 1/8 teaspoon iodized salt
- 1 tablespoon butter
- 2 medium peeled, thinly sliced peaches 3
- lightly beaten organic eggs

Preparation:

1. Preheat oven to 400 °F. Toss peaches and raspberries with sugar in a container.

2. Melt butter in a 9-inch round baking plate. Mix eggs, milk, plus salt in a small bowl until blended; whisk in the flour.

3. Remove the round baking plate from the oven, tilt to coat

the bottom and sides with the melted butter; pour in the flour mixture.

4.In the oven, bake until it becomes brownish and puffed. Remove the pancake from the oven. Serve immediately with more raspberries and vanilla yogurt.

Nutritional info:

Calories 199, Sodium 173 mg, Carbohydrates 25 g, Proteins 9 g, Sugar 11 g, Fibres 3 g, Fats 7 g

87

TURKEY & BEANS LETTUCE WRAPS

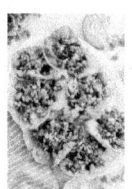

Preparation Time: 15 Minutes

Cooking Time: 13 Minutes

Serves: 4

Ingredients:
- 8 large butter lettuce leaves
- ¼ C. onion, minced
- 1/8 tsp. ground cumin
- Freshly ground black pepper, to taste
- 1 C. tomato, chopped
- 4 oz. lean ground turkey
- 2 garlic cloves, minced
- 2 tsp. olive oil
- 1/3 C. cooked black beans
- 3 tbsp. avocado, peeled, pitted, and chopped

Preparation

1. In a large container of chilled water, add lettuce leaves and set aside until serving.

2. In another container, add turkey, onion, garlic, and cumin and mix until well combined. In a large skillet, heat oil over medium heat.

3. Add turkey mixture and cook for about 8-10 minutes.

4. Stir in beans and tomato and reduce the heat to low. Cook for about 2-3 minutes and remove from heat. Set aside to cool.

5. Remove lettuce leaves from water and pat dry gently with a paper towel. Palace lettuce leaves onto plates. Top with remaining 4 leaves.

6. Divide turkey mixture onto each doubled lettuce leaves evenly.

7. Top with avocado pieces. Roll lettuce leaves to cover the turkey mixture and serve immediately.

Nutritional info:

Calories: 217, Fat: 11.8g, Carbohydrates: 14.5g, Fibre: 5g, Sugar: 3.3g, Protein: 15.2g, Sodium: 26mg

88

BANANA BREAD

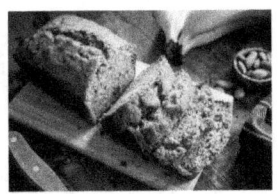

Preparation Time: 15 Minutes
Cooking Time: 60 Minutes
Servings: 14
Ingredients:
- Vegetable oil cooking spray
- ½ cup brown rice flour
- ½ cup amaranth flour
- ½ cup tapioca flour
- ½ cup millet flour
- ½ cup quinoa flour
- ½ cup of raw sugar
- ¾ cup egg whites
- 1/8 teaspoon iodized salt
- 1 teaspoon baking soda
- 2 tablespoons grapeseed oil
- 2 pieces of mashed banana

Preparation:
1. Preheat oven to 350 °F. Coat a loaf pan with a vegetable oil cooking spray, dust evenly with a bit of flour, and set aside.

2. In a container, mix the brown rice flour, amaranth flour, tapioca flour, millet flour, quinoa flour, and baking soda.

3. Coat a separate container with vegetable oil, then mix eggs, sugar, and mashed bananas.

4. Pour the bowl of wet fixing into the bowl of dry fixing and mix thoroughly. Scoop the mixture into the loaf pan. Bake within an hour.

5. To check the doneness, insert a toothpick in the centre of the loaf pan; if you remove the toothpick and it has no batter sticking to it, remove the bread from the oven.

6. Slice and serve immediately and store the remaining banana bread in a refrigerator to prolong shelf life.

Nutritional info:

Calories 150, Sodium 150 mg, Fibres 2 g, Sugar 7 g, Proteins 4 g, Fats 3 g

89

POACHED PEARS

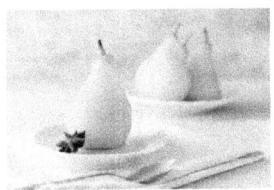

Preparation Time: 15 Minutes
Cooking Time: 30 Minutes
Servings: 4
Ingredients:
- ¼ cup apple juice extract
- 2 cup of orange juice extract
- 1 teaspoon cinnamon, ground
- 1 teaspoon ground nutmeg
- 1 tablespoon orange zest
- 4 whole pears, peeled, destemmed, core removed

Preparation:

1. In a container, combine the fruit juices, nutmeg, and cinnamon, and then stir evenly.

2. In a shallow pan, pour the fruit juice mixture, and set to medium fire.

3. Adjust the heat to simmer within 30 minutes; turn pears frequently to maintain poaching, do not boil.

4. Transfer poached pears to a serving container; garnish with orange zest and raspberries.

Nutritional info:
Calories 140, Fats 0.5 g, Carbohydrates 34 g, Proteins 1 g, Fibres 2 g, Sodium 9 mg

90

STRAWBERRY BRUSCHETTA

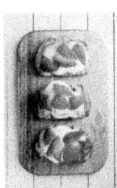

Preparation Time: 15 Minutes

Cooking Time: 0 Minutes

Servings: 12

Ingredients:
- 1 loaf sliced Ciabatta bread
- 5 tablespoons balsamic glaze
- 2 containers of strawberries, sliced
- 1 cup basil leaves
- 8 ounces goat cheese

Preparation

1. Wash and slice strawberries; set aside.
2. Rinse and chop the basil leaves; set aside.
3. Slice the ciabatta bread and spread some goat cheese evenly on each slice; add strawberries, balsamic glaze, and top with basil leaves.
4. Serve on a platter.

Nutritional Info

Calories 80, Sodium 59 mg, Fats 2 g, Proteins 3 g, Carbohydrates 12 g

CONCLUSION

At first glance, the DASH Diet may seem like one of those fad diets on TV that make grand promises about how easy it is to lose weight. And according to many, the DASH diet certainly qualifies. It is advertised as being so easy that "even your grandmother can do it".

The DASH diet, also known as the DASH (Dietary Approaches to Stop Hypertension) diet, was developed by a team of doctors, nutritionists, and healthcare professionals at the National Heart, Lung and Blood Institute.

The DASH diet was intended to lower blood pressure and reduce the risk of heart disease by eating a high intake of fruits, vegetables, and low-fat dairy foods.

The DASH diet is often mischaracterized as being a "so-called" diet that includes foods like soda, crackers, candy bars, and chips. Those foods are all part of the DASH diet, but consuming them is not necessary to follow the DASH diet.

The DASH diet can be used as a tool to manage blood pressure, and it's great for people who want to lose weight, but it is not really designed to help you lose weight. This diet is planned only for those who already have hypertension and seek a way to

Conclusion

lower their blood pressure. It's important to note that many people who have tried the DASH diet have found it challenging to stick with.

In all likelihood, you will not lose weight if you follow the DASH diet because it was not designed to help you lose weight. Experts warn that nutritionists and healthcare professionals unfamiliar with this diet may recommend it as a weight loss plan that could cause problems for some people. The DASH diet is also not intended to be an all-inclusive guide for healthy eating, and it would be wise to consult with your doctor and a nutritionist before starting this diet.

Here's another interesting fact about the DASH diet: many people who have tried this diet report that they feel better on it. One of the main benefits of following a heart-healthy diet is that it seems to benefit people's brains in addition to their hearts.

Finally, this complete guide to the DASH diet empowers you to eat all the foods you love as long as they come in a healthy package. This is not a "diet" but rather it's a way of life. It's not about following rules or even about weight loss--it's about living an active and satisfying life with food that tastes good and is good for you.

www.ingramcontent.com/pod-product-compliance
Lightning Source LLC
Chambersburg PA
CBHW071622080526
44588CB00010B/1234